THE INVERTED MEDICAL DICTIONARY

Second Edition

Mary J. Stanaszek, R.R.A.
Medical Record Administrator, Norman, Oklahoma

Walter F. Stanaszek, Ph.D.
Professor of Pharmacy Practice, College of Pharmacy, University of Oklahoma, Oklahoma City, Oklahoma

Bruce C. Carlstedt, Ph.D.
Associate Professor of Pharmacy Practice, School of Pharmacy & Pharmacal Sciences, Purdue University, West Lafayette, Indiana

Steven Strauss, Ph.D.
Professor of Pharmacy Administration, Arnold & Marie Schwartz College of Pharmacy and Health Sciences, Long Island University, Brooklyn, New York

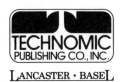

TECHNOMIC
PUBLISHING CO., INC.

LANCASTER · BASEL

The Inverted Medical Dictionary
a **TECHNOMIC**®publication

Published in the Western Hemisphere by
Technomic Publishing Company, Inc.
851 New Holland Avenue
Box 3535
Lancaster, Pennsylvania 17604 U.S.A.

Distributed in the Rest of the World by
Technomic Publishing AG

Printed in the United States of America
10 9 8 7 6 5 4 3 2 1

Main entry under title:
  The Inverted Medical Dictionary

A Technomic Publishing Company book
Bibliography: p.

Library of Congress Card No. 90-65013
ISBN No. 87762-825-4

HOW TO ORDER THIS BOOK

BY PHONE: 800-233-9936 or 717-291-5609, 8AM–5PM Eastern Time

BY FAX: 717-295-4538

BY MAIL: Order Department
Technomic Publishing Company, Inc.
851 New Holland Avenue, Box 3535
Lancaster, PA 17604, U.S.A.

BY CREDIT CARD: American Express, VISA, MasterCard

CONTENTS

PREFACE

Just as medicine is an extremely complicated science, so is its terminology. The ability to quickly find the proper medical term for any specific situation is, therefore, an undeniable asset to anyone engaged in the health care professions or involved with its literature. When the correct term is known, its definition can easily be found in a standard medical dictionary. However, when the meaning or situation is apparent but the proper medical term must be defined, the same dictionary is of little assistance.

A wide variety of medical terms, encompassing the basic or general foundations of medical terminology and terms reflective of current health care practice are listed herein. For this reason, both eponyms and medical abbreviations are also included. Some obsolete medical terms have been added because they are still occasionally found in the literature. The headings under which terms are presented were selected as those likely to be most obvious to the reader, and generally reflect either the subject or its most descriptive word. Many unclassified phrases are listed under two or more headings.

A number of additional sections have been compiled to assist the reader in use of this basic guide to the medical literature. These include drug and chemical abbreviations, terms used in prescription writing, weight and measure equivalents, and several anatomical illustrations.

ALPHABETICAL LISTING
OF TERMS

abdomen, upper part
midriff

abdominal cavity distension
celiectasia

abdominal fluid
ascites

abdominal fissure
hologastroschisis
a narrow opening or crack of considerable length and depth

abdominal gas
tympanism
swelling of the abdominal area due to intestinal gas

abdominal incision
celiotomy
a cut into the abdominal cavity
laparotomy
through the loin or flank

abdominal pain
formen
severe griping or colicky pain

abdominal wall suture
celiorrhaphy
laparorrhaphy

abnormal blood pressure
dysarteriotony

abnormal development
teratogenesis

abnormal formation
cacogenesia
cacogenesis

abnormal sensation
paresthesia
as of burning, prickling, or tingling

abnormal sense of taste
dysgeusia

abnormal size of head
macrocephalia
macrocephaly

abnormal sweating
diaphoresis

abnormal thirst
anadipsia
dipsosis

abnormal tissue development
dysplasia

abortion
embryotocia

absence of anatomical parts
agenesis
organ or part

(development)
agnathia
lower jaw
amastia
mammary glands
amelia
limbs
amyelia
spinal cord
anandria
male characteristics
anephrogenesis
kidney tissue
anorchism
testes
apneumia
lungs
apodia
feet
aprosopia
face
arhinia
nose
asternia
sternum
atrichosis
hair

3

absence of life
abiosis

absence of menstruation
amenorrhea

absence of pleasure
anhedonia
　　from acts that would otherwise be pleasurable

absorbent
desiccant
exsiccant

acetone bodies in blood
acetonemia

Achilles tendon pain
achillodynia

Achilles tendon suture
achillorrhaphy

acid, excessive
acidosis
　　in body fluids
supersalt
　　in salt

acid measurer
acidimeter

acidity deficiency
hypoacidity

activity deficiency
hypopraxia

"Adam's apple"
prominentia laryngea
　　prominent area in front of the neck

adenoids inflammation
adenoiditis

adenoids knife
adenomatome
　　surgical instrument for cutting adenoids
adenotome
　　surgical instrument for cutting a gland or adenoids

adenoids excision
adenoidectomy

after intercourse
postcoital

after surgery
postoperative

after vaccination
postvaccinal

air bacteria collector
aerobioscope
　　device to determine bacterial content in the air

air-breathed measurer
aeroplethysmograph
　　instrument to measure the amount of air breathed out (exhaled)

air dust measurer
aeroscope
　　instrument used in determining the purity of the air
konometer
　　instrument for counting the number of dust particles in the air

air/gas anywhere in body
pneumatosis
　　in any abnormal location

air/gas in brain ventricles
pneumocranium
pneumocephalus

air/gas in heart chambers
pneumatocardia

air/gas in intestines
aerenterectasia
meteorism
tympanites
　　also in abdomen

air/gas in joints
pneumarthrosis

air/gas in peritoneal cavity
aeroperitoneum
aeroperitonia

air/gas in pleural cavity
pneumothorax

air/gas in skull
epidural aerocele
usually caused by fracture

air/gas in spinal canal
pneumorrhachis

air/gas under the skin
pneumoderma
subcutaneous emphysema

air/gas in urine
pneumaturia

air/gas vaginal distention
aerocolpos

air in heart
aerendocardia

air-inspired measurer
inspirometer
instrument to measure the force, frequency, or volume of inhaled air

air in mediastinal tissues
pneumomediastinum

air in pericardial sac
pneumohydropericardium

air/saliva swallowing
aerosialophagy
sialoaerophagy
entry of of air and saliva into the stomach

air swallowing
aerophagia
aerophagy

air/water treatment
aerohydropathy
aerohydrotherapy

albumin measurer
albuminometer
instrument to measure albumin contents, especially in the urine

albumin in urine
albuminuria
noctalbuminuria
excess albumin in urine passed at night

alcohol in urine
alcoholuria

alertness of mind
eunoia

alimentary canal
enteron

alimentary canal lacking
agastric .

alkalinity in blood
alkalemia

alkalinity in urine
alkalinuria

allergic disease
allergosis
any disease resulting from allergy

allergic reaction
atopy
specifically with strong familial tendencies

allergic skin disorder
allergodermia

altered hematin in urine
urohematin
urofuscohematin
red pigment in urine

altitude sickness
Acousta's disease

ambisexual
hermaphroditism
hermaphrodism
condition of having both ovarian & testicular tissue

amebas in urine
ameburia

amines in urine
aminuria

amino acids in blood
aminoacidemia
presence of the enzyme in excessive amounts

amino acids in urine
   acidaminuria
   aminoaciduria

ammonia compounds in blood
   ammoniemia

ammonia in urine
   ammoniuria

amnion inflammation
   amnionitis

amnion lacking
   anamnionic
   anamniotic
      without the membrane normally surrounding the fetus

amnion ruptured
   amniorrhexis

amnion fluid escaped
   amniorrhea

amount desired
   ad lib (ad libitum)
      as desired

anatomy study
   morphology
      study of the structure and forms of organisms

anesthesia below waist
   para-anesthesia
      affecting only the lower half of the body

anesthesia by cold
   cryanesthesia
   refrigeration anesthesia

anesthesia by electricity
   electroanalgesia
   electronarcosis
      insensitivity to pain by use of electrical current

anesthetic measurer
   anesthesimeter

aneurysm repair
   aneurysmoplasty
   arterioplasty

aneurysm suture
   aneurysmorrhaphy

aneurysm of vein/artery
   phlebangioma
   phlebarteriectasia

angel dust
   phencyclidine (PCP)
      "street drug" subject to abuse

angle measurer
   goniometer

animal anatomy
   zootomy

animal breeding
   zoogony

animals, collectively
   fauna

antibody producer
   antigen
      anything that produces antibodies

antimony poisoning
   stibialism

antrum (sinus) operation
   antrostomy
   antrotomy
      opening of the antrum for drainage purposes
   antrectomy
      excision of the antrum

anus aperture lacking
   aproctia

anus artificial
   colostomy
      creation of an artificial anus in the abdominal wall by surgical means

anus inflammation
   periproctitis
   perirectitis
      inflammation of the connecting tissues around the rectum or anus
   proctitis
   rectitis
      inflammation of the rectum or anus

anus inflammation (cont.)
sphincteritis
inflammation of the anal sphincter muscle

anus pain
proctagra
proctalgia
proctodynia
proctalgia fugax
sphincteralgia

anus proximity
perianal
surrounding the anus

anus specialist
proctologist
physician who specializes in treating anal conditions

anus stricture
proctostenosis

anus viewer
anoscope
instrument to examine anus and rectum

aorta inflammation
aortitis
mesaortitis
inflammation of the middle layer of the aorta
periaortitis
inflammation of the tissues surrounding the aorta

aorta membrane
endaortitis

apathy
ameleia
indifference

apex inflammation
apicitis
of a tooth root or a lung

aponeurosis inflammation
aponeurositis

aponeurotic operation
aponeurotomy

aponeurotic suture
aponeurorrhaphy

appendages
adnexa
anatomical parts that are cojoined

appendages of the eye
adnexa oculi
the lacrimal glands

appendages of the uterus
adnexa uteri
oviducts and ovaries

appendix inflammation
appendicitis

appendix operation
appendectomy

appetite in excess
bulimia

appetite lacking
anorexia

appetite unnatural
allotriophagy
pica
appetite for unusual or harmful substances
chthonophagia
chthonophagy
geophagy
desire to eat earth, clay, chalk, etc

application
epithem
anything placed on a wound or sore spot

arachnoid membrane inflamed
arachnitis

arm amputation
brachiotomy

arm lacking
monobrachius
congenital deformity

arm largeness
macrobrachia

arm pain
brachialgia

arm smallness
microbrachia

armless/headless
acephalobrachia
born without head and arms

armpit
axilla

aromatic urine
uraroma

arrow poison
curare
ukambin

arsenic treatment
arsenotherapy
use of arsenic agents to treat disease

arson compulsion
pyromania

arterial pressure low
hypopiesia

artery calcification
arteriostosis

artery calculus
arteriolith

artery constriction
arteriarctia
arteriostenosis

artery crusher
angiotribe
instrument for crushing an artery embedded in the tissue

artery degeneration
arteriasis
arteronecrosis

artery dilatation
arteriectasis
arteriomotor

artery disease
arteripathy

artery hardening
arteriosclerosis

artery inflammation
arteritis
exarteritis
of the outer layer
mesarteritis
of the middle layer
panarteritis
of all the arteries
periangitis
of outside tissues around an artery
periarteritis
of the outer layer and tissues surrounding an artery
polyangitis
perivasculitis
involving multiple blood vessels
stetharteritis
of the arteries of the thorax

artery narrowing
arteriostenosis
constriction or compression inhibiting the flow of blood

artery operation
arteriectomy
arteriotomy
arterioplasty

artery pressure measurer
hemadynamometer
instrument to measure the blood pressure within the arteries

artery rupture
arteriorrhexis

artery small
arteriole

artery spasm
arteriospasm

artery suture
arteriorrhaphy

artery twisting
arteriostrepsis
to stop a hemorrhage

artery/vein communicating
anastomosis

artery x-ray
arteriography

articulation difficulty
dyslalia

articulation inflamed
osteoarthritis
    degenerative disease of a joint

artificial anus
enteroproctia

artificial intelligence
computer reasoning

artificial substitution
prosthesis
    artificial parts to the body
prosthetist
    specialist in artificial substitution
prosthodontics
    branch of dentistry devoted to the resto-
    ration of teeth

asbestos inhaled
asbestosis

asexual reproduction
agamogenesis
agamogenetic
agamogony

astigmatism measurer
astigmatometer
astigmometer
    instrument to measure the extent of
    blurred and imperfect image due to im-
    perfect refraction

athlete's foot
dermatophytosis
tinea pedis

atmospheric humidity measurer
hygrometer
    instrument to measure moisture in the
    air

atmospheric study
meteorology

atomizer
nebulizer

atrophy diffuse
panatrophy
    of several parts

atrophy of skin
atrophoderma
    decrease in size or wasting away
atrophodermatosis
    of the cutis

attachment
bonding
    to object or person

attic operation
atticotomy
    opening of the tympanic attic

attraction
tropism
    involuntary attraction of an animal or
    vegetable organism toward a more de-
    sirable spot

attraction to corpses
necromania
    also desire for death

attraction/rejection of sun
heliotaxis
heliotropism
    phenomenon where plants or plant or-
    gans have a tendency to lean toward or
    away from the sun

autopsy
necropsy

aversion to food
anorexia nervosa
apocleisis
apositia

aviator's disease
aeroneurosis
    a nervous disorder

axes equal
homoaxial
homaxonial

B

bacilli in blood
bacillemia
  presence of a type of rod-shaped bacteria in the blood

bacilli in urine
bacilluria

back
dorsalis
  posterior

backing-up
regurgitation

backward bent
retroflexion

backward displacement
retroposition

bacteria in blood
bacteremia
endotoxemia

bacteria collector
aerobioscope

bacteria largeness
macrobacterium
megabacterium
  bacteria of unusually large size

bacteria study
bacteriology

bacteria in urine
bacteriuria

bad breath
halitosis
ozostomia
stomatodysodia
*bromopnea**
  *obsolete term

bad taste sensation
cacogeusia

bag of waters
amniotic sac

baldness (see hair loss)

ball-and-socket
enarthrosis
  such as knee joint

barber's itch
mentagra
sycosis

base of skull
basicranial

beaded hair
moniliform hair
  congenital disease of scalp

beast transformation
lycanthropy
  individual believes to be a wild beast

bedclothes plucking
carphology
floccillation

bedsore
decubitus ulcer

bedwetting
enuresis

before birth
antenatal
antepartum
prenatal
  the period of time preceeding birth

before death
ante mortem

behind the ear
postaurical

behind the eye
postocular

belching
eructation

belief of smaller body
micromania

belief of one's divinity
theomania

belief that one is a dog
cryanthropy

bend
geniculum
the bend in an organ

beryllium disease
berylliosis
lung disorder caused by exposure to fumes or dust particles of beryllium

between attacks
interictal
intercritical

between cartilages
intercartilaginous
interchondral

between cell divisions
interphase

between cells
intercellular

between eyelids
interpalpebral

between lobes
interlobar
between the projecting parts of an organ or other structure

between muscles
intermuscular

between nostrils
internarial

between nuclear layers
internuclear
of the retina

between parietal bones
interparietal
also between the walls of any cavity

between ribs
intercostal

between similar structures
interspace

between teeth
interdentium
interdental
interocclusal

between thighs
interfemoral

between two adjoining surfaces
interproximal

bile duct dilation
cholangiectasis

bile duct inflammation
angiocholitis
cholangiolitiis
cholangitis
periangiocholitis
pericholangitis
inflammation of the tissues surrounding the bile ducts
pericholecystitis
inflammation around the gallbladder

bile duct operation
cholangiostomy
cholangiotomy

bile excessive formation
hypercholia

bile flow excessive
cholerrhagia
cholerrhagic
cholorrhea
hepatorrhea
polycholia

bile pigments
bilirubin
orange-red
biliverdin
green

bile secretion
choleresis
by liver

bile secretion lacking
acholia

bile in spinal fluid
bilirachia

bile in urine
biliuria
choluria

bilirubin in blood
bilirubinemia
hyperbilirubinemia
excessive amounts in the blood

bilirubin in urine
bilirubinuria

birth control
contraception
contraceptive
prevention of contraception or impregnation by sperm

birth to males
androgenous

birth to one
monotocous

birthmark
nevus

biting self
autophagia
autophagy

black-and-blue marks
livedo
discolored patch on the skin

black-haired
melanotrichous

black sickness
kala-azar
a fatal infectious disease endemic in the tropics

black spot vision
scotodinia
dizziness with blurring of vision and headache

black tongue
melanoglossia

black urine
melanuria

black vomit
vomitus nigar

blackhead
comedo

blackness in organs
melanism
presence of black pigment in tissues, organs, and skin

bladder calculus
cystolithiasis

bladder/cervix
cervicovesical

bladder dilatation
cystectasia
cystectasy

bladder discharge
cystorrhea
mucous discharge from the bladder

bladder examination
cystoscopy
visual examination of the interior of the urinary bladder

bladder fissure
exstrophy
schistocystis

bladder hernia
cystocele
enterocystocele

bladder inflammation
cystitis
cystopyelitis
inflammation of bladder and pelvis of the kidneys
paracystitis
pericystitis
epicystitis
inflammation of connecting tissues around the bladder

bladder inflammation (cont.)
 pyelocystitis
  inflammation of the bladder and pelvis of
  a kidney
 trigonitis
  inflammation of the trigone
 cystoureteritis
  inflammmation of bladder and ureters

bladder lacking
 acystia
  born without urinary bladder

bladder operation
 cystectomy
 cystotomy
 epicystotomy
 vesicotomy
 cystolithectomy
 cystolithotomy
  removal of calculi from urinary bladder
 cystopexy
  fixation of bladder
 cystoplasty
 cystollytroplasty
 cystoproctostomy
 cystostomy
 neocystostomy
 proctocystoplasty
 vesicostomy
  repair to the bladder
 ureteroileoneocystostomy
  a segment of the ileum is made part of
  the ureter

bladder pain
 cystalgia

bladder paralysis
 acystinervia
 cystoplegia

bladder prolapse
 cystoptosis
  the slipping of the urinary bladder from
  its normal position

bladder proximity
 paracystic
 paravesical

bladder tool
 bilabe
  used in removing foreign matters
  through the urethra
 cystometer
  instrument to study pressure and capac-
  ity of the bladder

 cystourethroscope
  instrument to examine posterior urethra
  & bladder

bladder x-ray
 cystography
 cystourethrography

bleeding after delivery
 postpartum hemorrhage

bleeding arrester
 hemostat
  an agent/instrument that stops bleeding

blind spot
 scotoma
  within the visual field

blindness
 amaurosis
 amaurotic
 typhylosis
 amaruosis fugax
  temporary blindness
 amblyopia
  dimness of vision
 hemeralopia
  day blindness
 hemianopsia
  blindness in half of visual field
 meropia
  partial blindness
 quadrantanopia
 quadrantanopsia
  loss of vision in one fourth of visual field

blister causing
 epispastic
 vesicant

blister groups
 herpetiform

blistering disease
pemphigus
   various types of skin diseases

bloodw/acetone
acetonemia
   in relatively large amounts

blood albumin low

hypoalbuminemia
hypoalbuminosis

blood alkalinity increased
alkalemia

blood alkali measurer
hemoalkalimeter

blood w/ammonia compounds
ammoniemia

blood analysis
hemanalysis
   examination of the blood, especially by
   chemical methods

blood w/bacilli
bacillemia

blood w/bacteria
bacteremia

blood bilirubin excess
bilirubinemia
hyperbilirubinemia
   excessive amounts in the blood

blood in bone
hematosteon

blood calcium excess
calcemia
hypercalcemia

blood calcium low
hypocalcemia

blood carbon dioxide excess
hypercapnia
hypercarbia
   also increased arterial carbon dioxide
   tension

blood carotene excess
carotenemia

blood cell
hematocyte
hemocyte

blood cell disintegration
erythrocytolysis
hemocatheresis
hematocytolysis
hemocytolysis
hemocytotripsis
hemolysis
   the alteration, dissolution or destruction
   of red blood cells, caused by a specific
   agent, toxicity or change in temperature.

blood cell formation
hematogenesis
hematopoiesis
hematosis
hemogenesis
hemopoiesis

blood cell measurer
erythrocytometer
hemocytometer

blood chloride low
hypochloremia

blood w/chyle
chylemia
   presence of chyle in the circulating
   blood

blood/chyle in urine
hematochyluria

blood clot
embolus
hematoma
thrombus

blood clot destruction
thromboclasis
thrombolysis

blood clot operation
embolectomy
thrombectomy
   surgical removal

blood clotting agent
prothrombin

blood coagulation disorder
coagulopathy
any disorder
consumptive coagulopathy
disseminated intravascular coagulation

blood w/cystine
cystinemia

blood deficiency
hyphemia
ischemia
oligemia

blood w/diacetic acid
diacetemia

blood disease
dyscrasia
hemopathy

blood disease study
hematopathology

blood drinking
hematophagia

blood elements low
hypocythemia
deficiency of red blood cells

blood w/epinephrine
adrenalinemia
adrenemia

blood w/fat excess
hyperlipemia
hyperlipidemia
hyperlipoidemia
lipemia
lipidemia
lipoidemia
presence of an abnormally large amount
of lipids in the blood

blood w/fibrin
fibremia
fibrinemia

blood filtration
hemofiltration
removal of waste products by passing
the blood through a filter

blood flow
hemokinesis
hemorrhage

blood flow arrest
electrohemostasis
hemostasia
hemostasis
arrest of circulation in a body part or
stagnation of blood

blood flow measurer
flowmeter
hemadrometer
hemadromometer
hemodromometer
hemotachometer
rotameter

blood fluid deficiency
anhydremia
hemoconcentration

blood fluid increase
hemodilution

blood formation
hematopoiesis

blood w/foreign matter
embolemia
usually blood clots

blood formation defective
anhematopoietic
anhematosis

blood freezing point
hemocryoscopy
process of determining the freezing
point of blood

blood gas measurer
aerotonometer

blood w/glucose
euglycemia
glycemia

blood w/glucose (cont.)
  hyperglycemia
    excessive amounts

blood w/gonococci
  gonococcemia

blood hemorrhage
  hematorrhea

blood w/heparin
  heparinemia

blood w/inositol
  inosemia

blood w/insulin
  insulinemia
    excessive amounts

blood iron low
  hypoferremia

blood in joint
  hemarthrosis

blood w/ketone bodies
  ketonemia

blood lacking alkali
  acidosis
    decrease of alkali in proportion to the acid

blood lacking hemoglobin
  oligochromemia

blood lacking lymphocytes
  alymphocytosis
  lymphopenia

blood w/lactic acid excess
  lactacidemia

blood leukocytes deficient
  leukopenia

blood measurement
  hematometry
    used to determine the number and types of cells, formed elements or hemoglobin present

blood w/melanin
  melanemia

blood w/methemoglobin
  methemoglobinemia

blood w/nitrogen
  azotemia
  hyperazotemia
  uremia
    excessive amounts

blood oxalates in excess
  oxalemia

blood oxygen low
  hypoxemia

blood phosphates high
  hyperphosphatemia

blood phosphates low
  hypophosphatemia

blood plasma low
  apoplasmia

blood platelets low
  thrombocytopenia
  thrombopenia

blood w/pneumococci
  pneumococcemia

blood w/poikilocytes
  poikilocythemia
  poikilocytosis

blood poisoning
  toxemia
  toxicemia
    poisoning in general
  radiotoxemia
    poisoning induced by overexposure to radioactive substances
  scatemia
    poisoning through the intestine

blood w/polypeptides
  polypeptidemia

blood potassium elevated
  hyperkalemia
  hyperpotassemia

blood potassium low
hypokalemia
hypopotassemia

blood pressure
arteriotomy

blood pressure elevated
hypertension

blood pressure estimator
hemomanometer

blood pressure low
hypotension

blood pressure measurer
sphygmotonometer
sphygmo-oscillometer
sphygmomanometer
   instrument to measure arterial blood
   pressure
ochrometer
   measures capillary pressure

blood protein high
hyperproteinemia
proteinemia

blood protein low
hypoproteinemia

blood prothrombin low
hypoprothrombinemia
prothrombinopenia

blood recycling
hemodialysis
   by diffusion through a semipermeable
   membrane

blood relationship
consanguinity

blood in semen
hematospermatocele

blood sodium elevated
hypernatremia

blood sodium low
hyponatremia

blood speed measurer
rheometer
   instrument to measure the velocity of
   blood current
stromuhr
   instrument to measure the speed of
   blood flow within blood vessels

blood in spinal cord
hematomyelia

blood w/sodium
natremia
natriemia

blood specialist
hematologist

blood spitting
hemoptysis

blood stone
hemolith

blood in stool
hematochezia
   passage of bloody stools

blood study
hematology
hematopathology
hemodiagnosis
hemodynamics
hemorrheology

blood substitute
periston

blood w/sugar
glycemia
hyperglycemia
   excessive amounts

blood sugar lacking
aglycemia

blood transfusion
autotransfusion
   transfusion of one's own blood

blood in tympanic cavity
hematotympanum
hemotympanum

blood w/uric acid
uratemia
uricacidemia
uricemia
hyperuricemia
excessive amounts

blood in urine
hematocyturia
natriemia

blood w/urobilin
urobilinemia

blood in uterus
hematometra
hematosalpinx
in uterine tube

blood in vagina
hematocolpos

blood vessel calculi
angiolith

blood vessel constriction
vasoconstriction

blood vessel development
angiogenesis

blood vessel dilatation
angiotelectasia
angiotelectasis
hemangiectasia
hemangiectasis
phlebarteriectasia
vasodilation

blood vessel enlargement
angiomegaly
increase in size of blood vessels or lymphatics

blood vessel formation
angiopoiesis

blood vessel hardening
angiosclerosis

blood vessel inflammed
angiotitis
endangitis
endangeitis

blood vessel inflammed (cont.)
endarteritis
inflammation of the blood vessels of the ear
endovasculitis
endophlebitis
generally inflammation of the intima of a blood vessel
endaortitis
endoartitis
inflammation of the aorta

blood vessel narrowing
angiostenosis

blood vessel nutritional disorder
angiodystrophia
angiodystrophy

blood vessel oozing
angiostaxis

blood vessel operation
angioneurectomy
angioplasty
angiorrhaphy
angiostomy
angiotomy

blood vessel paralysis
angioparalysis
angioparesis

blood vessel rupture
angiorrhexis
rhexis
rupture of a blood vessel or lymphatic

blood vessel spasm
angiospasm
angiospastic

blood vessel tumor
angioma
hemangioma
swelling from proliferation of the vessel

blood w/virus
viremia

blood volume high
hypervolemia

blood volume low
hypovolemia

blood vomiting
hematemesis

blood without sugar
aglycemia
aglycemic

blower
insufflator
instrument used to blow air, gas, water, etc. into a body cavity

blue blood
cyanemia

blue hands/feet
acrocyanosis

blue skin
cyanochroic
cyanochrous
cyanoderma
cyanosis

blue sweat
cyanephidrosis
cyanhidrosis
excretion of sweat with a bluish tint

boat-shaped
scaphoid

boat-shaped head
cymbocephaly
scaphocephaly

body curve measurer
cyrtometer

body deformity correction
orthopraxis

body dryness
xerotes

body in excess
polysomia
polysomus
developmental anomaly with doubling or tripling of the body size

body largeness
gigantism
macrosomia

body measurer
anthropometer
instrument used for measurements of thebody
anthropometrist
operator of the instrument
anthropometry
art of measuring the body

body odor
bromhidrosis
bromidrosis
bromohyperhidrosis

body pain
pantalgia

body smallness
dwarfism
microsomia
nanism
nanosomia
meromicrosomia
smallness of some body parts

body temperature low
hypothermia
hypothermy

body type
somatotype
constitutional or body type of an individual

boil
furuncle
an abscess

bone
os
ossa

bone cell
osteoblast

bone cutter
osteotome
osteotribe
rongeur

bone death/decay
osteolysis
osteonecrosis
decay in general
osteoradionecrosis
caused by radiation

bone development
osteogenesis

bone development defective
anostosis
osteodystrophy

bone disease
osteochrondrosis
osteopathia
osteopathology
osteopathy
osteopoikilosis

bone enlargement
hyperostosis

bone formation
osteosis

bone formation defective
dysostosis
osteochondrodystrophia
disorder of bone and cartilage formation

bone hemorrhage
osteorrhagia

bone hardening
osteosclerosis

bone inflammation
osteitis
osteoarthritis
bone and joint
osteochrondritis
bone and cartilage
osteomyelitis
bone marrow
osteosynovitis
bone and synovial membrane
osteophlebitis
veins of a bone
osteoperiostitis
bone and periosteum

bone inflammation (cont.)
panosteitis
entire bone
periostitis
petrositis
fibrous membrane covering part of the temperol bone

bone knife
osteotome

bone marrow inflammation
medulitis
medullitis
myelitis
osteomyelitis

bone marrow tumor
myeloma
composed of cells derived from hemo-poietic tissues of the bone marrow

bone measurement
osteometry

bone/membrane adhesion
meningosis
as in the skull of the newborn

bone nutrition
osteotrophy

bone operation
ostearthrotomy
ostectomy
osteoarthrotomy
osteoclasis
osteoplasty
osteorrhaphy
osteostixis
osteotomy

bone pain
ostalgia
ostealgia
osteocope
osteodynia
osteoneuralgia

bone regeneration
osteanagenesis

20

bone regeneration (cont.)
osteanaphysis
reproduction of bone

bone in skin
osteodermia

bone softening
halisteresis
osteomalacia
osteoporosis

bone specialist
orthopedist
physician specializing in diagnosis and
treatment of the skeletal system

bone study
orthopedics
osteology

bone suppuration
ostempyesis
pus in the bone

bone suture
osteorrhaphy
osteosuture

bone tumor
osteocarcinoma
osteochondrofibroma
osteochondroma
osteochondrophyte
osteoclastoma
osteocystoma
osteofibroma
osteoma
osteonucus
osteophyma
osteosarcoma
osteospongioma

border
limbus

both sides
ambilateral

bowels uncontrollable
scatacratia
scoracratia
incontinence of feces

brain
encephalic
encephalon

brain abscess
encephalopyosis

brain atrophy
encephalatrophy

brain calculus
encephalolith

brain disease
encephalosis
organic disease
encephalomeningopathy
disease of brain and meninges

brain extract
sphingomyelin

brain gray matter
cinerea

brain hardness
cerebrosclerosis
encephalosclerosis

brain/head lacking
deranencephalia
born with neck, but no head or brain

brain hemorrhage
cerebral hemorrhage
encephalorrhagia

brain hernia
cephalocele
encephalocele
encephameningocele

brain imperfect
ateloencephalia

brain inflammation
cerebritis
encephalitis
ependymitis
the ependyma
ventriculitis
cerebral meningitis
cerebrospinal meningitis
myeloencephalitis

brain inflammation (cont.)
meningitis
meningocephalitis
meningoencephalitis
   brain and spinal cord
meningocerebritis
   brain and meninges
meningoencephalomyelitis
   meninges, brain and spinal cord
mesencephalitis
   midbrain
periencephalitis
poliencephalitis
   surface of the brain
polioencephalitis
   gray matter of the brain
polioencephalomeningomyelitis
   gray matter of the brain and spinal cord
   meninges
polioencephalomyelitis
poliomyelitis
   gray matter of the brain and spinal cord

brain knife
encephalotome
   instrument used in brain surgery

brain lacking
anencephaly
pantanencephalia
pantanencephaly

brain largeness
macrencephaly
macrencephalous

brain operation
encephalotomy
leukotomy
lobotomy
topectomy
ventriculostomy
ventriculotomy

brain puncture
encephalopuncture
ventriculopuncture
   puncture of the brain substance

brain pus
encephalopyrosis
pyencephalus

brain smallness
micrencephalia
micrencephaly
micrencephalous
microencephaly
   abnormal smallness in size of the brain

brain softness
cerebromalacia
encephalodialysis
encephalomalacia

brain/spinal cord disease
encephalomyelopathy
encephalomyeloradiculopathy

brain/spinal cord inflammation
arachnoiditis
encephalomyelitis

brain/spinal cord lacking
amyelencephalia
amyelencephalus
amyelencephalous
amyelencephalic
amyelia
amyelic
amyelous
amyelus
   congenital absence

brain stone
encephalolith
   a calculus (stone) in the brain or one of
   its ventricles

brain tissue hardening
sclerencephalia
sclerencephaly

brain tumor
encephaloma
glioma
meningioma

brain x-ray
encephalogram

breast atrophy
  mastatrophy
  mastatrophagia

breast disease
  mastopathy
    any abnormal condition of the breast

breast excess number
  pleomastia
  pleomazia
  pleomaziax
  polymazia

breast hemorrhage
  mastorrhagia

breast inflammation
  mastitis
  paramastitis
  perimastitis
    tissues around the breast

breast largeness
  macromastia
  macromazia
  mammose
  mastauxe

breast operation
  mammectomy
  mammoplasty
  mastectomy
  mastopexy
  mastoplasty
  mastotomy

breast pain
  mammalgia
  mastalgia
  mastodynia
  mazodynia

breast smallness
  micromazia
    rudimentary presence only

breast tumor
  mastoderma
  mastochondroma

breath odor
  halitosis
  ozostomia
  ozostomiax
  bromopnea*
    **obsolete term

breathing absence
  apnea

breathing difficulty
  atelectasis
  dyspnea

breathing fast
  tachypnea

breathing machine
  respirator

breathing slowness
  bradypnea

breathing sound
  rale
  rhonchus
    diagnosed during examination

bronchi inflammation
  bronchadenitis
    bronchial lymph nodes
  bronchiolitis
    bronchioles
  bronchitis
    bronchial tubes
  bronchopneumonia
  bronchopneumonitis
    bronchi and lungs
  peribronchitis
  peribronchiolitis
    tissues surrounding thebronchi/
    bronchioles

bronchial calculus
  broncholith
    the calculus (stone)
  broncholithiasis
    the medical condition

bronchial dilation
  bronchocele

bronchial fistulization
bronchostomy
through the chest wall

bronchial suture
bronchorrhaphy

bronchial viewer
bronchoscope

bruise
contusion

bunion
hallux valgus
deviation of main axis of the great toe

bunion operation
bunionectomy

burning pain
causalgia
persistent severe burning sensation of the skin

bursa inflammation
bursitis

bursa operation
bursectomy

buttocks pain
pygalgia

buttocks pertaining
gluteal

buttocks too fat
steatopygia

bypass
shunt

C

calcified fetus
lithokelyphopedion
lithokelyphopedium

calcified fetus (cont.)
lithopedion
lithopedium
osteopedion*
*obsolete term

calcium antagonist
calcium channel blocker
slow channel blocker

calcium in bile
calcibilia

calcium in blood
calcemia
hypercalcemia
excessive amount
hypocalcemia
abnormally low levels

calcium lacking in diet
calciprivia

calcium regulation
calmodulin
protein present in all nucleated cells

calcium in tissues
calcinosis

calcium in urine
calciuria
hypercalcinuria
hypercalciuria
hypercalcuria

calculi destroying
electrolithotrity
disintegration of calculi (stones) in the urinary bladder

calculi formation
calciphylaxis
calculosis
lithiasis
lithogenesis

calculi smallness
microlithiasis
microlith

calf-bone
fibula

24

callosity
heloma durum
hard corn
helome molle
soft corn

callus
tyloma

callus formation
tylosis

camphor poisoning
camphorism

cancer
carcinoma
sarcoma
(see also tumor under specific site)

cancer dissemination
carcinolytic
carcinomatosis
carcinosis
metastasis

cancer formation
carcinogenic
carcinogenesis
causing cancer

cancer specialist
cancerologist
oncologist

cancer study
cancerology
oncology
cynodont
a tooth having one cusp or point

capillary dilation
capillarectasia
telangiectasia
trichangiectasia
obsolete term

capillary disease
capillaropathy
telangiectasia

capillary inflammation
capillaritis

capsule inflammation
capsulitis

capsule instrument
capsulotome
cystotome
surgical instrument for incising the capsule of a lens with cataract

capsule operation
capsulectomy
capsulotomy
capsuloplasty

capsule suture
capsulorrhaphy

carbohydrates in urine
carbohydraturia

carbolic acid in urine
carboluria

carbon compounds in urine
carbonuria

carbon dioxide in blood
hypercapnia
hypercarbia
excessive amounts
hypocapnia
hypocarbia
abnormally low tension of carbon dioxide

carbon dioxide measurer
carbonometer
obsolete device

carbon dust disease
anthracosis

carotene in blood
carotenemia
excessive amounts

carpal bone operation
carpectomy

cartilage cell
chondrocyte

cartilage disease
chondropathy

cartilage formation
chondrogenesis
chondroplasia
chondroplasia

cartilage hardening
chondrocalcinosis

cartilage inflammaiton
chondritis
general term
meniscitis
inflammation of the semilunar cartilage
of the knee joint
perichondritis
inflammation of the perichondrium

cartilage knife
arthrotome
chondrome

cartilage operation
chondrectomy
chondroplasty
chondrotomy
meniscectomy
on the semilunar cartilage
thyrochondrotomy
thyrotomy
on the thyroid cartilage

cartilage pain
chondralgia
chondrodynia
chondrodynia
xyphodynia

cartilage softening
chondromalacia
softening of any cartilage

cartilage tumor
chondroadenoma
chondroangioma
chondroblastoma
chondrofibroma
chondrolipoma
chondroma
chondromyoma
chondromyxoma
chondromyxosarcoma

cartilage tumor (cont.)
chondrosarcoma
chondrosteoma

casts in urine
cylindruria
presence of renal cylinders or casts in
the urine

cataract
phacomalacia
phacosclerosis
sclerocataract
obsolete term

cataract operation
phacocystectomy
phacoerysis

cat's whiskers
vibrissa
applies to hair in the nose

cecum calculi
typhlolithiasis

cecum dilatation/distention
typhlectasis

cecum enlargement
typhlomegaly

cecum hernia
cecocele
typhlocele*
*obsolete term

cecum inflammation
cecitis
typhlenteritis
typhlitis
typhlodicliditis
inflammation of the iliocecal valve

cecum operation
cecectomy
cecotomy
cecostomy
typhlectomy
typhlostomy

cecum suture
cecorrhaphy

cell counter
cytometer
glass slide or chamber used in counting and measuring

cell deficiency
cytopenia

cell death
necrocytosis

cell destroyer
cytocele
cytoclasis
cytotoxic

cell development
cytogenesis

cell dissolution
cytolysis

cell division
mitosis

cell fusion
plasmatogamy
plasmogamy
plastogamy
union of two or more cells with preservation of the individual nuclei

cell granulation
emiocytosis
exocytosis
release of secretory granules or droplets from a cell

cell largeness
macrocyte

cell membrane
plasmalemma

cell-produced poison
endotoxin

cell repair
cytothesis
repair of injury to cells

cell rupture
erythrocytorrhexis
plasmorrhexis

cell size equal
isocellular

cell smallness
microcyte

cell stimulus
cytropism
tendency of cells to move toward or away from stimuli

cell study
cytogenetics
cytology

cerebellum lacking
notanencephalia
born without cerebellum

cerebral convolutions lack
agyria
born without cerebral convolutions

cerebral hemispheres fused
cyclencephalia
cyclencephaly
cyclocephalia
cyclocephaly

cerebrospinal
encephalorrhachidian

cerebrospinal sugar
glycorrhachia
in the fluid
hyperglycorrhachia
excessive amounts

cerebrum/cerebellum lacking
anencephalia
anencephaly

cerum excess
ceruminosis

cervix/bladder
cervicovesical

cervix inflammation
cervicitis
trachelitis
cervicocolpitis
cervix and vagina

cervix operation

cervicectomy

trachelectomy

trachelopexy

tracheloplasty

trachelotomy

trachelorrhaphy

Cesarean birth

partus caesarius

change

metamorphosis
in form, structure or function

change of life

climacteric

menopause

cheek

bucca

mala

cheek cleft

meloschisis
congenital condition

cheek inflammation

melitis
general term
gnathitis
also of the jaw

cheek pertaining

malar
cheek or zygoma
buccogingival
cheek and gums
buccolabial
cheek and lip
buccolingual
cheek and tongue
buccopharyngeal
cheek and pharynx

cheekbone

os zygomaticum

cheeselike

tyroid

chemical attraction

chemotaxis
property of cells to be attracted to or re-
pelled by chemical stimuli

chemical breakdown

catabolism
often accompanied by the liberation of
energy

chemical change

metabolism

chest

pectus

thorax
especially the anterior wall

chest deformity

thoracococyllosis

thoracocyrtosis

thoracogastroschisis

thoracomelus

thoracoschisis

chest disease

thoracopathy

chest examination

stethoscopy
by means of listening to the cardiac and
respiratory sounds

chest measurement

stethogoniometer

stethometer

thoracometer

chest narrowness

stenothorax

thoracostenosis

chest pain

stethalgia

thoracalgia

thoracodynia

thoracomyodynia

chest operation

thoracectomy

thoracentesis

thoracolysis

thoracoplasty

chest operation (cont.)
thoracopneumoplasty
thoracostomy
thoracotomy

chest spasm
stethospasm

chewing
mastication

chewing incomplete
psomophagia
psomophagy

chewing force measurer
phagodynamometer
instrument to measure the force exerted

chicken breast
pectus carinatum
prominence of the sternum

chickenpox
varicella

childbearing
texis

childbirth
tocus
tokus
oxytocia
oxytocic

childbirth dry
xerotocia

childbirth normal
eutocia

childbirth psychosis
tocomania
postpartum psychosis

childbirth study
obstetrics
tocology

children perversion
pedophilia
sexual perversion

children physician
pediatrician
pediatrist

children study
pediatrics

chill of death
algor mortis

chin/lip
labiomental

chin operation
genioplasty

chin smallness
microgenia

chlorides in blood
hyperchloremia
high levels
hypochloremia
low levels

chlorides in urine
chloriduria
chloruresis
hyperchloruria
high levels
hypochloruria
low levels

cholesterol in blood
cholesteremia
cholesterolemia
hypercholesterolemia
excessive amounts
hypocholesteremia
low levels

cholesterol in tissues
cholesterosis
cholesterolosis

cholesterol in urine
cholesteroluria

choroid inflammation
choroiditis
general term
choroidocyclitis
choroid and ciliary processes

29

choroid inflammation (cont.)
chorioretinitis
choroid and retina

chronaxie measurer
chronaximeter

chyle in blood
chylemia

chyle deficiency
achymia
hypochylia
oligochylia

chyle in excess
hyperchylia
polychylia

chyle forming
chylifacient
chyliferous

chyle lacking
achylia
achylous
absence of normal intestinal fluid produced during digestion

chyle in pericardium
chylopericardium

chyle in peritoneum
chyloperitoneum

chyle/lymph in urine
chyluria

ciliary body destruction
cyclodiathermy

ciliary body inflamed
cyclitis
general term
cyclochoroiditis
ciliary body and choroid

ciliary body knife
cyclotome

ciliary body operation
cyclectomy
cyclodialysis
cyclotomy

ciliary muscle paralysis
cycloplegia
cycloplegic
pertaining to muscles surrounding the
eyeball

ciliary operation
ciliarotomy
zonulotomy

cirrhosis of liver
hepatocirrhosis

clap
gonorrhea

clavicle operation
clavicotomy

clavicle/sternum angle
sternoclavical angle

cleft extremity
schistomelus
individual with one or more cleft limbs

cleft face
schistoprosopus

cleft palate
palatoschisis
palatum fissum

cleft tongue
schistoglossia
congenital fissure of the tongue

clitoris enlargement
clitoromegaly

clitoris inflamed
clitoriditis
clitoritis

clitoris operation
clitoridectomy
clitoridotomy
clitoroplasty

clotting
coagulation
changing from liquid to solid or solid to
gel

clotting (cont.)
electrocoagulation
using an electric current

cloudiness measurer
turbidimeter
instrument for determining the extent of cloudiness in a liquid

clubfoot
talipes equinovarus

clubhand
talipomanus

clumsy with either hand
ambilevous
ambisinister

clustered
agminate
agminated

clusterlike
botryoid
racemose

coccyx operation
coccygectomy

coccyx pain
coccyalgia
coccygodynia

coexistence
mutualism
symbiosis
living together of organisms of different species for common advantage

coin-shaped
mummiform
mummular

coitus climax unreached
anorgasmy

coitus interrupted
coitus interruptus
onanism

coke
cocaine

cold
algid

cold anesthesia
cryanesthesia

cold pain
cryalgesia
psychralgia
pain produced by application of cold

cold sensitiveness
cryesthesia
hypercryalgesia
hypercryesthesia

cold sore
herpes simplex

cold/warm sensation
psychroesthesia
feeling of cold in warm parts of the body and of warmth in cold parts

colon disease
enteromycosis
enteropathogenesis
enteropathy

colon distention
pneumocolon

colon inflammation
colitis
general term
mucocolitis
mucous membranes
paracolitis
outer tissues of the colon
enterocolitis
enteritis
small intestine and colon
perisigmoiditis
sigmoiditis
sigmoid fold of the colon
coloproctitis
colorectitis
proctocolitis
rectum and colon
proctosigmoiditis
rectum and sigmoid colon

colon inflammation (cont.)
rectocolitis
    rectum membrane & colon

colon largeness
megacolon
macrosigmoid
megasigmoid
    sigmoid colon

colon operation
colectomy
colotomy
enterocentesis
enterocolectomy
enterocolostomy
enteroenterostomy
enterolysis
enteropexy
enteroplasty
hemicolectomy
lumbocolostomy
lumbocolotomy
pancolectomy
rectosigmoidectomy
sigmoidectomy
sigmoidotomy
sigmoidopexy
sigmoidoproctostomy
sigmoidorectostomy
sigmoidosigmoidostomy
typhlostomy
typhlotomy
ureterocolostomy
ureteroenterostomy
ureterosigmoidostomy

colon smallness
microcolon
    often arising from a decreased function-
    al state

colon suture
colorrhaphy

color blindness
achromate
    the individual
achromatopsia
    general term

color blindness (cont.)
daltonism
    red-green
color amblyopia
    partial
cyanopia
cyanopsia
    all objects appear blue
deuteranopia
    red
dyschromatope
    difficulty distinguishing colors
monoblepsia
monochromasy
monochromatism
monochromatic
    only one color perceived
protanomaly
protanopia
    defective red vision
xanthocyanopsia
    yellow and blue visible, not red

color blindness detector
anomaloscope
leukoscope

color intensity measurer
chromatometer
colorimeter

color normal
normochromic

colored cell
chromocyte

colored sweat
chromhidrosis

colorless cell
achroacyte

column of liquid curve
meniscus
    the curved surface of a column of liquid

compression
tamponade

compulsive touching
phaneromania

concave skull
clinocephaly
   condition where the top of the head is saddle-shaped

concentration lacking
aprosexia

conduct study
praxiology

condyle operation
condylectomy
condylotomy

conflicting mental forces
ambivalence

conjunctiva dryness
xerophthalmia

conjunctiva inflammation
conjunctivitis
blepharoconjunctivitis
   conjunctiva & eyelids

conjunctiva mucous flow
ophthalmoblenorrhea

conjunctiva operation
conjunctivoplasty
logadectomy
peritectomy
peritomy

conjunctiva patch
pinguecula
   a whitish spot on the conjunctiva

conjunctiva tumor
conjunctivoma

conjunctiva varicosity
varicula
   swelling of the veins of the conjunctiva

convulsion
paroxysm

coordination defective
hyposynergia
chalcosis

cord operation
chordotomy

cord operation (cont.)
cordectomy
cordotomy
   surgical procedure on the spinal cord

corn
clavus
heloma

corn surgery
helotomy

cornea curve measurement
keratometry

cornea disease
keratopathy

cornea with fat
corneal steatosis
lipoidosis corneae

cornea growth
keratoma
keratosis

cornea inflammation
keratitis
   general term
keratoconjunctivitis
   cornea and conjunctiva
keratoiritis
   cornea and iris
keratoscleritis
sclerokeratitis
   cornea and sclera
sclerokeratoiritis
   cornea, sclera, and iris

cornea inspection
keratoscopy

cornea knife
keratome
keratotome
   surgical instrument used to cut into the cornea

cornea largeness
macrocornia
megalocornea

cornea opaque ring
arcus cornealis
arcus juvenilis
arcus lipoides
arcus senilis

cornea operation
keratectomy
keratoleptynsis
keratophakia
keratoplasty
keratotomy
kerectomy

cornea outer layer
ectocornea

cornea protrusion
keratectasia
keratoconus
keratoglobus

cornea puncture
keratocentesis
keratonyxis

cornea rupture
keratorrhexis
due to trauma or perforating ulcer

cornea/sclera bulging
staphyloma
staphylomatous

cornea smallness
microcoria
microcornea

cornea softness
keratomalacia
due to disease or Vitamin A deficiency

cornea spot
albugo
leukoma
walleye

cornea ulcer
keratohelcosis
ulcus serpens

cornea viewer
keratoscope

corpulence
adiposis
obesity

cotton-mill fever
byssinosis

cough
tussis

counting inability
anarithmia

crack
cocaine

cranial gas/air
erpidural aerocele
accumulation of gas or air in the skull, usually after a fracture

cranial hernia
hydrencephalocele
hydrencephalomeningocele
notencephalocele
notencephalus

cranial knife
craniotome
instrument used to perforate the fetal skull

cranial operation
cephalocentesis
craniotomy

cranial pressure measurer
cephalohemometer

craving
parepithymia
abnormal longing

crib death
sudden infant death syndrome

critical stage
acme

crosslike
cruciform

croup
laryngitis

crystals in urine
crystalluria

cup-shaped
scyphiform
schyphoid

curvature of spine
kyphosis
hunch back
lordosis
leaning backward
scoliosis
lateral curvature

cut
laceration

D

daily recurrence
quotidian

dandruff
dermatitis seborrheica
furfur
pityriasis capitus

"dandruff of the gods"
cocaine

dark vision
scieropia
defective vision with objects appearing dark

darkness measurer
biophotometer
instrument for measuring adaptation to darkness

darnel poisoning
loliism

day blindness
hemeralopia

deafness
anacusis
anakusis

death apparent
anabiosis
anabiotic
involves resuscitation; also used to denote an agent utilized in restoring life

death chill
algor mortis

death by electrocution
electrothanasia

death without pain
euthanasia

decline of disease/fever
catabasis
paracme

decomposition by light
photolysis

deep stained cell
chromatophil
chromophil

deep voice
baryphonia

deer fly fever
tularemia

defecation painful
dyschezia

defective fusion
araphia
dypraphia
dysraphism
holorachiochisis
spina bifida of the spinal column

deficiency of amniotic fluid
oligohydramnios

deficiency of bile
oligocholia

35

deficiency of blood
oligemia
oligocythemia
oligoplasmia

deficiency of chyle
oligochylia
lack of sufficient digestive fluid

deficiency of hair
hypotrichosis
oligotrichia

deficiency of hemoglobin
oligochromemia
in the blood

deficiency of menstruation
oligomenorrhea
reduction in frequency

deficiency of milk secretion
oligogalactia

deficiency of nutrition
oligotrophia
oligotrophy

deficiency of oxygen
hypoxemia
in the blood

deficiency of phosphates
oligophosphaturia
in the urine

deficiency of saliva
oligoptyalism
oligosialia

deficiency of sodium
hyponatremia
in the blood

deficiency of sperm
oligospermia
oligozoospermia

deficiency of teeth
oligodontia

deficiency of thirst
oligodipsia
abnormal absence of thirst

deficiency of urine
oliguria

deformity generalized
pantamorphia

deformity straightening
orthosis
orthotic

degeneration
retroplasia
decreased cell activity associated with injury or death

delusion of greatness
megalomania
megalomanic

dental enamel formation
amelification

dentistry
gerodontics
for the elderly
odontology
orthodontics
dental orthopedics
pedodontics
for children

dentition painful
dysodontiasis

depilatory
epilation

depression
melancholia

descent
matrilineal
through the female side
patrilineal
through the male side

designer drugs
street drugs
substance abuse

desire for confinement
claustrophilia

desire for music
melomania

desire to steal
kleptomania

desquamation
ecdysis
casting off of the outer skin

deterioration mental
dementia
due to organic or psychological factor

determining by touch
topesthesia

development of disease
pathogenesis

development incomplete
agenesia
agenetic
agenesis
aplasia

dextrose in urine
*dextrosuria**
glycosuria
*obsolete term

diacetic acid in blood
diacetemia

diacetic acid in urine
diacetonuria
diaceturia

diaphragm inflammation
diaphragmitis

diarrhea astringent
albumin tannate

diarrhea of food
lientery
undigested food is evacuated

diastole lacking
adiastole

dietary fiber
cellulose
roughage

dietary treatment
alimentotherapy
dietotherapy
sitotherapy

dietetics
sitiology
sitology

difference in color
heterochromia
heterochromous
between two structures or parts that are normally similar

difference in origin
heterogeneous

differs from normal form
heteromorphous

difficulty in articulation
dysarthria
dyslalia

difficulty in coordination
dyspraxia
dystaxia
dyssynergia

difficulty in defecation
dyschezia

difficulty in speech
dyslogia
dysphasia
dysphonia
dysphrasia
resulting from cortical damage

difficulty in standing
dystasia

difficulty in swallowing
dysphagia
odynophagia

difficulty in teething
dysodontiasis

difficulty in urination
dysuria

difficulty in walking
dysbasia

digitalin-like
apocynein
a glycoside from dogbane with the effect of digitalin

digits fused/lacking
ectrosyndactyl

dilatation of artery
aneurysm

dilatation of heart
cardiectasis

dilator
speculum
instrument to create an opening

dirt/clay eating
geophagia
geophagy
geophagism
geophagist
individual who eats

discharge suppression
ischesis
retention of discharge or secretion

discomfort
dysphonia
feeling of unpleasantness or discomfort

disease of .....
see under specific location

disease classification study
nosology
nosotaxy

disk inflammation
discitis
diskitis

displacement forward
anteversion
anteverted

dog-head shaped
cynocephalus

dosage determination
dosimetry

dosage study
posology
the science of dosage

double chin
buccula

double clitoris/penis
diphallus

double eyelashes
distichiasis

double hearing
diplacusis

double joint
diarthric
relating to two joints

double lip
dicheilia
dichilia

double pupil
dicoria
diplocoria
discoria
presence of a double pupil in the eye

double uterus
didelphia
dimetria

double vision
amphodiplopia
diplopia
monodiplopia

dream analysis
oneiroscopy

drinkable
potable

drop
gutta
abbreviated as ggt and refers to drop of medication (i.e., eye drops)

dropsy of abdomen
ascites

dropsy of the brain
hydrocephalus
retention of fluid

drug action
pharmacodynamics
pharmacology

drug-disease study
pharmacotherapeutics

drug fondness
pharmacomania

drug holiday
drug withdrawal
for brief period during treatment

drug study
biopharmaceutics
pharmacodynamics
pharmacoepidemiology
pharmacology
pharmacognosy

drug treatment
chemotherapy
pharmacotherapy
treatment of disease by means of chemical substances or drugs

drug use multiple
polypharmacy
use of many products simultaneously

drunkard nose
rhinophyma

dry
siccus

dryness
xerotes

dry childbirth
xerotocia
dry labor

dry mouth
xerostomia

dry nasal passages
xeromycteria
extreme dryness of mucous membrane

dry skin
xeroderma
xeronosus
xerosis

drying agent
desiccant

drying out
exsiccation

ductus deferens operation
vasectomy
vasoepididymostomy
vasoligation
vaso-orchidostomy
vasostomy
vasotomy
vasovasostomy
vasovesiculectomy

dullness of intellect
asynesia
asynesis
hebetude
lack of easy comprehension and practical intelligence

dumping syndrome
gastric emptying

duodenum inflammation
duodenitis
periduodenitis
tissues around the duodenum

duodenum operation
duodenectomy
duodenotomy
duodenocholecystostomy
duodenocystostomy
duodenocholedochotomy
duodenoenterostomy
duodenojejunostomy
pancreatoduodenectomy
duodenostomy

duodenum suture
duodenorrhaphy

duodenum x-ray
duodenogram

dura mater
pachymeninx
    outer membrane of the brain

dura mater disease
pachymeningopathy

dura mater inflammation
pachymeningitis
perimeningitis
peripachymeningitis

dura mater operation
duraplasty

dwarf
nanus
nanous

dwarfism
nanism

E

ear damaging
ototoxic
    having a toxic action upon the ear

ear deformity
otocephaly

ear disease
otopathy
otosclerosis
tympanosclerosis

ears excessive
polyotia
    born with more than two ears

ear hairs
tragal

ear hemorrhage
othemorrhagia
otorrhagia

ear implant
auditory prosthesis
cochleal prosthesis

ear inflammation
barotitis
otitis
otoantritis
otomycosis
otopyosis
panotitis
perilabyrinthitis
    inner ear
pyolabyrinthitis
    labyrinth with pus
tympanitis
    eardrum
tympanomastoiditis
    eardrum and mastoid cells

ear largeness
macrotia

ear mucous discharge
otopyorrhea
otopyosis
otorrhea

ear murmuring
syrigmus

ear-nose-throat specialist
otorhinolaryngologist

ear-throat study
otolaryngology

ear operation
myringotomy
ossiculectomy
ossiculotomy
otoplasty
ototomy
stapedectomy
stapediotenotomy
tympanectomy
tympanoplasty
tympanotomy

ear operation (cont.)
vestibulotomy

ear-originated
otogenic
otogenous

ear external lacking
anotia

ear polyp
otopolypus

ear purulent drainage
otopyorrhea

ear smallness
microtia

ear study
otology
otolaryngology
ears and throat
otoneurology
includes nerves
otorhinolaryngology
ears, nose, and throat
otorhinology
ears and nose

ear thickness
pachyotia

ear tube
cochlea
organ of hearing in the central ear

ear viewer
otoscope

eararache
otalgia
otodynia
otoneuralgia

eardrum
tympanic membrane

eardrum infection
mycomyringitis
myringomycosis

earth eating
geophagia

earth eating (cont.)
geophagism
geophagy
geophagist
individual involved

earthworm
lumbricus

earthworm-like
lumbricoid

eating animal food
carnivorous
zoophagous

eating aversion
apocleisis

eating in excess
polyphagia
bulimia
hyperphagia
binge eating caused by mental disorder

eating fast
tachyphagia

eating one food
monophagism
habit of subsisting on one type of food

eggwhite-like
glairy

eighth day fever
octan fever

elbow
cubitus

elbow disease/deformity
cubitus valgus
cubitus varus
olecranarthropathy

elbow inflammation
olecranarthritis
olecranarthrocace

elevation
torulus

embryo development
embryogenesis

41

embryo development (cont.)
embryogeny
   period of about the third to ninth week of
   pregnancy

embryo disorder
embryopathy

embryo nutrition
embryotrophy

embryo operation
embryectomy
embryotomy
embryoctony

embryo study
embryology

EMG syndrome
exomphalos, macroglossia, and gigantism
   also known as Beckwith-Wiedemann
   syndrome

endocardium inflamed
endocarditis

enlargement of ...
   see under specific organ

entrance
introitus

epididymis inflamed
epididymitis
epididymo-orchitis
   epididymis and testis

epididymis operation
epididymectomy
epididymotomy
epididymovasostomy

epigastric hernia
epigastrocele
   hernia in the epigastric region

epigastrium pain
epigastralgia

epiglottis inflamed
epiglottis
   area at the root of the tongue

epiglottis operation
epiglottidectomy

epinephrine in blood
adrenalinemia

epinephrine in urine
adrenalinuria

epiploon/omentum lacking
anepiploic

equal axes
homaxial

equal form
homeomorphous

equilibrium
homeostasis
   state of balance in the body functions

erection persistent
priapism

erector muscle
arrector
   a muscle that raises

erotic ecstasy
nympholepsy

erythrocytes color variation
anisochromasia

erythrocyte deficiency
oligocythemia

erythrocytes unequal
anisocytosis

esophagus dilatation
esophagectasia
esophagectasis
megaesophagus

esophagus distention
esophagocele
   protrusion of the membrane through a
   tear in the muscular coat

esophagus examination
esophagoscopy

esophagus inflamed
esophagitis

esophagus operation
esophagectomy
esophagocoloplasty
esophagomyotomy
esophagoplasty
esophagotomy
esophagoenterostomy
esophagojejunostomy
esophagoesophagostomy
esophagogastrectomy
esophagogastroplasty
esophagogastrostomy
esophagostomy
esophagotomy

esophagus pain
esophagalgia
esophagodynia

esophagus prolapse
esophagoptosia
esophagoptosis

esophagus spasm
esophagism
causing difficulty in swallowing

esophagus stricture
esophagostenosis

esophagus/stomach viewer
esophagoscope

etiology unknown
agnogenic
cryptogenic

evacuation involuntary
scatacratia
scoracratia
incontinence of feces

evacuation opening abnormal
allochezia
allochetia

evil spirit possession
cacodemonomania
belief of possession

excessive acid
acidosis
in blood or urine

excessive activity
hyperanakinesia

excessive hunger
sitomania

exciting heart action
cardiokinetic

exhale/inhale measurer
spirometer
instrument used to measure respiratory
gases

expansion
rarefaction
process of becoming light or less dense

expectorating pus
pyoptysis

external ear
auris externa

extrauterine gestation
metacyesis
ectopic pregnancy

extremity cleft
schistomelus

extremity cold
acrohypothermy

extremity clubbing
acropathy

extremity lacking
acolous
amelia
amelus

extremity pain
melagra

extremity pertaining
acral

extremity senseless
acroanesthesia
lack of feeling

eye
oculus
ophthalmus

eye acuteness equal
isopia

eye adhesion
syncanthus

eye angle study
gonioscopy
examination of the angle of the anterior
chamber of the eye

eye appendages
adnexa oculi

eye choroid hernia
choriocele

eye crossed
convergent strabismus
esotropia

eye discharge
ophthalmorrhea

eye disease
ophthalmopathy
any pathologic condition

eye fluid
aqueous humor

eye fusion
cyclopia
cyclops
synophthalmus

eye hemorrhage
ophthalmorrhagia

eye images equal
isoiconia

eye inflammation
canthitis
canthus of the eye
choroiditis
choroid layer
conjunctivitis
conjunctiva
ophthalmia
ophthalmitis
general term
ophthalmomyitis
eye muscles

eye inflammation (cont.)
ophthalmoneuritis
ophthalmic nerve
panophthalmia
panophthalmitis
entire structure
papilloretinitis
optic disk and retina
parophthalmia
near the eye
scleritis
sclerotitis
sclera
sclerochoroiditis
scleroticochoroiditis
choroid and sclera
scleroiritis
sclera and iris
sclerokeratitis
sclera and cornea
sclerokeratoiritis
sclera, cornea, and iris
xenophthalmia
conjunctiva

eye lacking
anophthalmia
anophthalmos
anophthalmus

eye largeness
buphthalmos
megalophthalmus
megophthalmus

eye layers
choroid
middle, vascular layer
retina
inner layer
sclera
outer layer

eye malformation
cryptophthalmia
cryptophthalmos
cryptophthalmus
congenital deformity

eye mechanical
ophthalmotrope

eye muscle balance
orthophoria
normal condition

eye muscle measurer
optomyometer

eye nerve paralysis
ophthalmoplegia
paralysis of the motor nerves of the eye

eye ointment
oculentum

eye operation
canthectomy
canthoplasty
canthotomy
canthorrhaphy
ophthalmomyotomy
ophthalmoplasty
ophthalmostasis
ophthalmotomy
orbitotomy
rhinommectomy
sclerectoirdectomy
sclerectomy
scleroplasty
sclerostomy
scleronyxis
sclerotomy
blepharoplasty
tarsectomy
tarsoplasty
tarsorrhaphy
tarsotomy

eye pain
ophthalmagra
ophthalmalgia
ophthalmodynia

eye pupil contracting
miosis

eye refraction measurer
refractometer
instrument used to measure the deflection of light rays

eye refraction unequal
anisometropia
heterometropia

eye shiny particles
synchysis scintillans
in the vitreous humor

eye softness
ophthalmomalacia
scleromalacia
synchysis
abnormal softening of the eyeball

eye specialist
oculist
ophthalmologist

eye steel detector
sideroscope
instrument used in detecting fragments of metal

eye tension measurer
tonometer

eye torsion measurer
clinoscope

eye turned left
levoversion
levoduction

eye turned right
dextroversion

eye turned upward
anaphoria
anatropia
habit or tendency

eye twitching
blepharospasm
blephaospasmus

eye viewer
auto-ophthalmoscope
ophthalmoscope

eyeball covering
conjunctiva
also coating inside the eyelid

eyeball dryness preventer
   antixerophthalmic
   antixerotic

eyeball enlargement
   buphthalmia
   buphthalmos
   buphthalmus

eyeball inflammation
   endophthalmitis
     inner tissues
   panophthalmitis
     all tissues
   trichiasis
   trichoma
     caused by misplaced eyelashes

eyeball measurer
   exophthalmometer
   exophthalmometry
   proptometer

eyeball movement
   oculogyration

eyeball protrusion
   exophthalmos
   exophthalmus
   ophthalmocele

eyeball recession
   enophthalmia
   enophthalmos
     recession of the eyeball within the orbit

eyeball rupture
   ophthalmorrhexis

eyeball smallness
   microphthalmia
   microphthalmus
   nanophthalmia
   nanophthalmos
   nanophthalmus

eyebrow loss
   madarosis

eyebrows meeting
   synophrys

eyebrow wrinkling
   ophryosis
     caused by spasmodic twitching of the nearby muscles

eyelash loss
   madarosis
   milphosis

eyelash excess
   polystichia
     more than one row

eyelid
   blepharon
   palpebra

eyelid adhesion
   ankyloblepharon
   blepharosynechia
   symblepharon

eyelid aperature small
   blepharophimosis

eyelid contraction
   blepharospasm
   blepharospasmus

eyelid/cornea adhesion
   corneoblepharon

eyelid drooping
   blepharoptosis

eyelid edema
   blepharedema
     causing a baggy appearance

eyelid growth
   xanthelasma

eyelid holder
   blepharostat
     speculum for diagnostic or treatment use

eyelid inflammation
   blepharitis
   palpebritis
   blepharadenitis
     tarsal glands
   blepharitis ciliari
   blepharitis marginalis

eyelid inflammation (cont.)
blepharoconjunctivitis
  fatty glands on the edge of the eyelids

eyelid inversion
entrophe
entropion

eyelid largeness
macroblepharia

eyelid not closing
blepharodiastasis
  abnormal separation or inability to close

eyelid operation
blepharectomy
blepharoplasty
blepharotomy
sphincterectomy

eyelid smallness
microblepharia
microblepharism
microblepharon

eyelid spasm
blepharoclonus

eyelid wink
nictate
nictation

eyelid suture
blepharorrhaphy
tarsorrhaphy

eyelid sweat
blepharochromhidrosis

eyelid softness
tarsomalacia
  of the cartilage

eyelid thickness
blepharopachynsis
pachyblepharon

eyelid tumor
blepharoadenoma
blepharoncus
blepharophyma

eyelid varicosity
varicoblepharon

eyelid wart
pladaroma
pladarosis
  a soft wartlike growth on the eyelid

eyestrain
copiopia

F

face cleft
schistoprosopus

face defective
prosoposchisis
  congenital fissure

face enlargement
pseudoacromegaly

face lacking
aprosopia
  congenital defect

face largeness
macroprosopia
megaprosopia
prosopectasia
macroprosopous
  the individual

face lift
rhytidoplasty

face narrowness
leptoprosopia

face/neck
cervicofacial

face pain
prosoponeuralgia

face shortness
brachyfacial
brachyprosopic

face smallness
microprosopus

face spasm
prosopospasm
risus sardonicus
  facial tic

facial neuralgia
prosopalgia
prosoponeuralgia
tic douloureux

facial paralysis
prosopoplegia
diplegia facial
prosopodiplegia

falling organ
prolapse
ptosis
blepharoptosis
  drooping of upper eyelid
gastroptosis
  falling of stomach
hysteroptosis
  falling of uterus

falling sickness
epilepsy

Fallopian tube calculus
salpingolithiasis

Fallopian tube hernia
salpingocele
salpingo-oophorocele

Fallopian tube inflamed
salpingitis
salpingo-oophoritis
  tubes and ovaries
salpingoperitonitis
  tubes and peritoneum

Fallopian tube operation
salpingectomy
salpingo-oophorectomy

Fallopian tube operation (cont.)
salpingoovariectomy
salpingopexy
salpingoplasty
salpingolysis
salpingostomatomy
salpingostomy
salpingotomy

Fallopian tube suture
salpingorrhaphy

Fallopian tube x-ray
salpingography

false anemia
pseudoanemia
  pallor of skin without signs of anemia

false joint
neoarthrosis
pseudarthrosis

false neuritis
pseudoneuritis

false pregnancy
phantom pregnancy
pseudocyesis

false ribs
costae spuriae

false smell
pseudosmia
  sensation of an odor that is not present

false taste perception
pseudogeusia

false tetanus
pseudotetanus

false vision
pseudoblepsia
pseudopsia
  visual hallucinations

farsightedness
hypermetropia
hyperopipresbyopia
presbyope

fascia inflammation
fascitis

fascia operation
fasiectomy
fascioplasty
fasciotomy
fasciodesis

fascia suture
aponeurorrhaphy
fasciorrhaphy

fast eating
tachyphagia

fast talking
agitolalia
agitophasia
tachylogia
tachyphasia
tachyphemia
tachyphrasia

fat
adipose
obese
pimelosis

fat absorption
lipometabolism
lipophagy
    ingestion of fat by a fat-absorbing cell

fat in blood
hyperlipemia
hyperlipidemia
lipemia
lipidemia
lipoidemia

fat cell
lipocyte

fat in cornea
lipoidosis corneae

fat decomposition
lipolysis
    chemical decomposition

fat decreasing
lipotropic

fat deficiency
lipopenia

fat deposits
adiposis
lipoidosis
lipomatosis
liposis
steatopygia
    in the cells

fat in feces
pimelorrhea
steatorrhea

fat formation/increase
lipogenesis
lipogenic
lipogenetic
lipogenous
lipotrophy

fat inflammation
pimelitis
    inflammation of adipose tissue

fat ingesting
ipophage

fat necrosis
steatonecrosis

fat particle
chylomicron
    microscopic particle occurring in chyle or
    blood

fat pertaining
aliphatic
sebaceous

fat resembling
lipoid

fat soluble
lipid
liposoluble

fat storing
adipopexis
adipopeptic

fat tumor
lipoma

fat tumor (cont.)
lipomyoma
lipomyxoma
liposarcoma
pimeloma
steatoma

fat in urine
adiposuria
lipiduria
lipoiduria
lipuria
    excretion of lipid in the urine

fat of wool
lanolin

Father of Medicine
Hippocrates
    Greek physician 460-377 B.C.

fatty degeneration
steatosis

fatty tumors
adiposis tuberosa simplex
Anders' disease
    nodular type, often on the abdomen

fauna and flora
biota

fear of air current
aerophobia

fear of alcoholic beverages
alcoholophobia

fear of angina pectoris
anginophobia

fear of animals
zoophobia

fear of bees
apiphobia
melissophobia

fear of being afraid
phobophobia

fear of being alone
monophobia
    morbid dread of solitude

fear of being beaten
rhabdophobia

fear of blushing
ereuthophobia

fear of books
bibliophobia
    morbid dread or hatred of books

fear to be bound
merinthophobia

fear of bridge crossing
gephyrophobia

fear to be buried alive
taphophobia

fear of cancer
cancerophobia
carcinophobia

fear of cats
ailurophobia

fear of certain places
topophobia

fear of change
neophobia
    morbid aversion to novelty or the un-
    known

fear of childbirth
maieusiophobia
tocophobia

fear of children
pedophobia

fear of choking
pnigophobia

fear of climbing
climacophobia

fear of closed places
claustrophobia

fear of cold
psychrophobia

fear of colors
chromatophobia
chromophobia

fear of confinement
claustrophobia

fear of contamination
mysophobia
fear of dirt or defilement from touching familiar objects

fear of crowds
ochlophobia

fear of dampness
hygrophobia

fear of darkness
nyctophobia
scotophobia
morbid fear of night or the dark

fear of dawn
eosophobia

fear of daylight
phengophobia

fear of death
necrophobia
thanatophobia

fear of deformity
taratophobia
in others
dysmorphophobia
in self

fear of depths
bathophobia

fear of deserted places
eremophobia
or of solitude

fear of dirt
mysophobia
rhypophobia

fear of disease
hypochondria
hypochondriasis
nosophobia
pathophobia

fear of dogs
cynophobia

fear of dolls
pediophobia
morbid fear aroused by the sight of a child or a doll

fear of draft/wind
aerophobia
anemophobia

fear of drugs
pharmacophobia

fear of dust
amathophobia

fear of eating
phagophobia
sitophobia

fear of electricity
electrophobia

fear of errors/sins
hamartophobia

fear of everything
panphobia

fear of fatigue
kopophobia
ponophobia

fear of feces
coprophobia

fear of fever
pyrexeophobia

fear of filth
rhypophobia
rupophobia

fear of fire
pyrophobia

fear of fish
ichthyophobia

fear of flashing light
selaphobia

fear of food
cibophobia
sitophobia
morbid fear of eating food

51

fear of forests
hylephobia

fear of fresh air
aerophobia
also of drafts

fear of frogs
batrachophobia

fear of fur
doraphobia
touching fur or skin

fear of germs
microphobia

fear of ghosts
phasmophobia

fear of glass
crystallophobia
hyalophobia

fear of God
heophobia

fear of hair
trichophobia
morbid disgust over loose hair
trichopathophobia
anxiety about one's hair

fear of hearing certain names
onomatophobia

fear of heart disease
cardiophobia

fear of heat
thermophobia

fear of heights
acrophobia

fear of hell
hadephobia
stygiophobia

fear to be home
ecophobia
oikophobia
fear of one's home surroundings

fear of humans
anthropophobia
phobanthropy

fear of ideas
ideophobia

fear of infection
molysmophobia

fear of injury
traumatophobia

fear of insanity
maniaphobia

fear of insects
entomophobia

fear of itching
acarophobia
also fear of parasites or of small particles

fear of jealousy
zelophobia

fear of left side
levophobia

fear of lice
pediculophobia

fear of light
photodysphoria
photophobia

fear of lightening/thunder
astrapophobia
keraunophobia

fear of loneliness
eremiophobia
eremophobia

fear of love
erotophobia
aversion to the thought of sexual love and expression

fear of machinery
mechanophobia

fear of many things
polyphobia

fear of marriage
gamophobia

fear of medicines
pharmacophobia

fear of men
androphobia
the male sex as a whole
anthropophobia
any man or men

fear of metal
metallophobia

fear of meteors
meteorophobia

fear of mirrors
spectrophobia

fear of missles
ballistophobia

fear of moisture/dampness
hygrophobia

fear of motion
kinesophobia

fear of naked persons
gymnophobia

fear of names
nomatophobia
onomatophobia

fear of needles
belonephobia
also of pins and other sharp pointed objects

fear of neglect
paralipophobia

fear of newness
neophobia

fear of night
nyctophobias
scotophobia

fear of nothing
pantaphobia
fearless

fear of novelties
neophobia

fear of odors
bromidosiphobia
osmophobia
osphresiophobia

fear of old age
gerontophobia

fear of open spaces
agoraphobia
cenophobia
kenophobia
also fear of leaving familiar surroundings

fear of own voice
phonophobia
or of any sound

fear of pain
algophobia

fear of parasites
acarophobia
parasitophobia
phthiriophobia

fear of people
anthropophobia

fear of personal uncleanliness
automysophobia

fear of personal odor
bromhidrosiphobia

fear of physical contact
aphephobia
haphephobia

fear of pins
belonephobia
or of any sharp pointed object

fear of places
topophobia

fear of pleasure
hedonophobia

fear of pointed objects
aichmophobia
fear of being touched by the object

fear of poison
iophobia
toxicophobia
toxiphobia

fear of poverty
peniaphobia

fear of prepices
cremnophobia

fear of pregnancy
maieusiophobia
extreme dread of childbirth

fear of projectiles/missles
ballistophobia

fear of rabies
lyssophobia

fear of railways
siderodromophobia

fear of rain
ombrophobia

fear of rectal disease
proctophobia
rectophobia

fear of red
erythrophobia

fear of religious/sacred objects
hierophobia

fear of responsibility
hypengyophobia

fear of returning home
nostophobia

fear of right side
dextrophobia
fear of objects to the right

fear of rivers
potamophobia

fear of robbers
harpaxophobia

fear of seas
thalassophobia

fear to be seen
scopophobia
a dread of being looked at

fear of self
autophobia

fear of sermons
homilophobia

fear of sexual intercourse
coitophobia
cypridophobia

fear of sexual love
erotophobia

fear of sharp objects
aichmophobia
belonephobia
as needles, pins, or any sharp object

fear of sins
hamartophobia
peccatiphobia

fear of sitting down
kathisophobia

fear of skin of animals
doraphobia

fear of skin diseases
dermatophobia

fear of sleep
hypnophobia

fear of small objects
microphobia
also fear of parasites or bacteria

fear of snakes
ophidiophobia

fear of society
anthropophobia
phobanthropy

fear of solitude
autophobia
eremophobia
monophobia

fear of sounds
acousticophobia
phonophobia

fear of speaking
laliophobia
morbid fear of speaking or stuttering

fear of spiders
arachnephobia

fear of stairs
climacophobia

fear of standing
stasiphobia
stasibasiphobia

fear of stealing
kleptophobia

fear of strangers
xenophobia

fear of streets
agyiophobia
a type of agarophobia

fear of stuttering
laliophobia

fear of sun rays
heliophobia

fear of syphilis
syphilophobia

fear of teeth
odontophobia

fear of thirteen
triakaidekaphobia
triskaidekaphobia
superstitious dread of the number thirteen

fear of thunder
astrapophobia
brontophobia
keraunophobia
tonitrophobia

fear of time
chronophobia

fear to be touched
aphephobia
haphephobia

fear of trains
siderodromophobia

fear of trauma
traumatophobia

fear of travel
hodophobia

fear of trembling
remophobia

fear of trichina
trichinophobia
fear of contracting disease from uncooked meat

fear of tuberculosis
phthisiophobia
tuberculophobia

fear of uncleanliness
automysophobia
fear of personal uncleanliness

fear of vaccination
vaccinophobia

fear of vehicles
amaxophobia
hamaxophobia
fear of meeting or of riding in any sort of vehicle

fear of venereal diseases
cypridophobia
venereophobia

fear of vomiting
emetophobia

fear of walking
basiphobia

fear of water
aquaphobia
potamophobia

fear of wind/draft
anemophobia

fear of women
> *gynephobia*

fear of work
> *ergasiophobia*
> *ponophobia*
>> aversion to work of any kind

fear of worms
> *helminthophobia*

fear of writing
> *graphophobia*

febrifuge
> *antipyretic*

febrile
> *pyrectic*
> *pyretic*

feces bag
> *colostomy bag*
>> also ileostomy bag

feces calcified
> *coprolith*
> *fecalith*

feces eating
> *coprophagy*
> *scatophagy*

feces with fat
> *pimelorrhea*
> *steatorrhea*
>> fatty diarrhea
>> excessive amounts

feces with pus
> *pyochezia*

feces uncontrolled
> *incontinence*

feeblemindedness
> *amentia*
> *cretinism*

feeding on carrion
> *necrophagous*
>> refers to decayed or decaying flesh

feeding on food of all kinds
> *omnivorous*

feeding on one food
> *monophagism*

feeding unnatural way
> *enteral feeding/nutrition*
> *hyperalimentation*
> *parenteral alimentation*
> *rectal alimentation*
>> forms of therapeutic nutritional intake

feeling of discomfort
> *dysphoria*

feeling of superiority
> *egomania*

feeling of well-being
> *euphoria*

feet in excess
> *polypodia*

feet gigantic
> *acrodolichmelia*
>> large size and disproportionate growth
>> of the hands and feet

feet lacking
> *apodia*
> *apodial*
> *apodous*
> *ectropody*
> *apody*
> *apus*
>> individual involved

feet largeness
> *macropodia*
> *megalopodia*
> *pes gigas*

feet malformed
> *peropus*

feet shortness
> *brachypodous*

feet sweat increased
> *acrohyperhidrosis*
>> also applicable to the hands

fertilization
> *gametogenesis*

fetal operation
>*amniotomy*
>*cephalotomy*

fetal surgical tool
>*cephalotome*
>*cephalotribe*

fetal thyroid tumor
>*microfollicular adenoma*

fetus calcified
>*lithokelyphopedion*
>*lithokelyphopedium*
>*lithopedion*
>*lithopedium*
>*osteopedion**
>>**obsolete term

fetus deformity
>*abrachiocephaly*
>*acephalobrachius*
>>without head and arms
>*acephalocardius*
>>without head and heart
>*acephalocheirus*
>*acephalochirus*
>>without head and hands
>*acephalogaster*
>>twin with pelvis and legs only
>*acephalopodius*
>>without head and feet
>*acephalorrhachia*
>>without head or vertebra
>*acephalostomia*
>>without head
>*acephalothorus*
>>without head and thorax
>*acephalus*
>>without head
>*acheilia*
>*achilia*
>>without lips
>*acheira*
>*achiria*
>>without hands
>*acorea*
>>without pupils
>*acormus*
>>without trunk

fetus deformity (cont.)
>*acrania*
>>without skull
>*acystia*
>>without urinary bladder
>*adactyl*
>>without fingers or toes
>*agenosomia*
>*agenosomus*
>>without genitalia
>*aglossia*
>>without tongue
>*aglossostomia*
>>without tongue or mouth opening
>*agnathia*
>>undeveloped or missing jaws
>*agyria*
>>without cerebral convolutions
>*amelia*
>*amelus*
>>without extremities
>*ametria*
>>without uterus
>*amyelencephalia*
>*amyelencephalus*
>>without brain and spinal cord
>*amyelia*
>*amyelic*
>*amyelous*
>*amyelus*
>>without spinal cord
>*anadidymus duplicatos*
>>pelvis and lower extremities united
>*aniridia*
>*irideremia*
>>iris lacking
>*anophthalmia*
>*anophthalmos*
>*anophthalmus*
>>without eyes
>*anorchia*
>>without testes
>*apleuria*
>>without ribs
>*apneumia*
>>without lungs
>*apodia*

fetus deformity (cont.)

apus
    without feet
aposthia
    without prepuce
aproctia
    without anus opening
aprosopia
    without face
arrhinia
arhinia
    without nose
asternia
    without sternum
astomia
    without mouth
atelencephalia
ateloencephalia
    with imperfect brain
athelia
    without nipple
atrachelocephalus
    head and neck missing or undeveloped
atresia
    imperforation of normal opening
atretocystia
    urinary bladder imperforate
atretogastria
    cardiac/pyloric orifice imperforate
brachycephalia
brachycephaly
    short head
brachychilia
    short lips
brachydactylia
brachydactlic
brachydactyly
    short fingers
brachyglossia
brachyglossal
    short tongue
brachygnathia
brachygnathous
    short lower jaw
brachykerkic
    forearm disproportionate
brachymetapody
    shortness of metatarsals or metacarpals

fetus deformity (cont.)

brachyphalangia
    shortness of phalanges
brachypodous
    short legs
brachyrhinia
    shortness of nose
brachyrhynchus
    shortness of maxilla and nose
brachyskelic
    short legs
abdominal fissure
celosomia
celosomus
schistocelia
schistocoelia
    open body with eventration
cryptophthalmos
    eyelids stuck together
cyclencephaly
cyclocephalia
cyclocephaly
    poor development of the two cerebral
    hemispheres
cyclopia
cyclops
    both eyes fused into one
deranencephalia
deranencephaly
    neck without head
didactylism
    only two fingers or toes
diglossia
    split tongue
dignathus
    two lower jaws
diphallus
    double penis
diplocoria
    double pupil
ectrodactylia
ectrodactyly
ectrodactylism
    fingers or toes missing
ectromelia
    limb missing or defective
ectropody
    without feet

fetus deformity (cont.)

ectrosyndactyly
   fingers/toes fused/lacking
hyperdactylia
hyperdactylism
hyperdactyly
polydactyly
   excessive fingers or toes
hypophalangism
   phalanges missing
hypospadias
   urethral opening abnormal
irideremia
aniridia
   iris lacking
lipostomy
   mouth missing
lithopedion
lithopedium
lithokelyphopedion
lithokelyphopedium
   calcified fetus
lusus naturae
   a monstrosity
melomelus
   rudimentary limb
melotia
   displacement of the ear
meroacrania
   parts of the skull missing
miopus
   additional rudimentary face
monobrachius
   having only one arm
monodactylism
monodactyly
   having only one finger or toe
monophthalmos
   having only one eye
monopidia
monopus
   having only one foot
monorchidism
monorchism
   having only one testis
omacephalus
   parasitic twin with imperfect head and
   no upper extremities

fetus deformity (cont.)

opocephalus
   without mouth and nose
ostembryon
   archaic term for lithopedion
otocephalus
   lower jaw missing
pantamorphia
   general deformity
pantanencephalia
pananencephaly
   without brain
paracephalus
   parasitic twin with defective head,
   trunks, and limbs
paragnathus
   parasitic fetus attached laterally to the
   jaw
peracephalus
   parasitic twin with only legs and pelvis
perobrachius
   forearms and hands malformed
perochirus
   hand absent or underdeveloped
perocormus
perosomus
   defective trunk
perodactylia
perodactyly
   fingers or toes defective
peromelia
peromelus
   malformation of limbs
peropus
   feet defective
perosomus
   body malformed
perosplanchnica
   viscera malformed
phocomelia
polymelus
   excessive number of limbs
polymeria
   additional body parts
polydentia
polyodontia
   excessive number of teeth
polyorchisism

fetus deformity (cont.)

polyorchism
polyorchis
  excessive number of testes
polyotia
  more than one ear
polyphalangia
polyphalangism
  additional phalanx in finger or toe
polypodia
  more than two feet
polythelia
  additional nipples
porencephalic
porencephalous
porencephaly
  insufficient development of the cerebral
  cortex and gray matter
proencephalus
  part of frontal skull missing
prognathism
  projecting jaws
pseudotruncus arteriosus
  defective heart and usually without pul-
  monary artery
ilioxiphopagus
  having two heads and two chests
schistocormus
  open thorax
schistoglossia
  cleft tongue
schistomelus
  cleft extremity
schistoprosopus
  fissue of the face
schistorrhachis
  open spinal cord
schistosomus
  lateral or middle eventration and defective lower extremities
schistosternia
  sternal fissure
schistothorax
  fissure of the thorax
schistotrachelus
tracheloschisis
  cervical fissure

fetus deformity (cont.)

schizogyria
  partial separation of the cerebral gyri
macropodia
  feet size excessive
symelus
symellus
sympus
  both legs fused together
sirenomelia
sirenomelus
sympus apus
uromelus
  fused legs and no feet
strophocephalus
strophocephaly
  deformity of lower face
sympus monopus
  fusion of legs with foot missing
cyclopia
synophthalmia
synophthalmus
  fusion of eyes and orbits
synorchidism
synorchism
  fusion of testes in the abdomen or scrotum
synotia
synotus
  union or near union of the ears in the
  neck region
tetrabrachius
  double fetus with four arms
tetradactyl
  four digits on each limb
tetramastia
  four breasts
tetrapus
tetrascelus
  four feet
tetramelus
  four legs or four arms
tetrastichiasis
  four rows of eyelashes
tetrotus
  four ears
thoracoceloschisis
  fissure of thorax and abdomen

fetus deformity (cont.)

thoracoschisis
fissure of thorax

tribrachius
three arms

tricephalus
three heads

triencephalus
triocephalus
no organs of sight, hearing or smell

triophthalmos
combined twins with three eyes

riopodymus
three faces with only one head

triorchidism
triorchis
three testes

triotus
three ears

hyperphalangism
triphalangia
triphalangism
three phalanges in the thumb or big toe

triprosopus
three faces fused into one

fetus first feces
meconium

fetus lacking
afetal

fetus monitor
cardiotography
monitoring of fetal heart rate

fetus nutrition
cyotrophy
embryotrophy

fetus ossified
lithopedion
ostembryon*
*obsolete term

fever blister
herpes simplex
herpes virus

fever causing
febrifacient
pyrogen

fever induced
hyperthermia

fever lacking
afebrile
apyrexia
apyrexial
apyretic

fever reducer
antipyretic

fibrin in blood
fibremia
fibrinemia
inosemia
presence in the blood, causing clotting

fibrocartilage inflamed
fibrochondritis
inochondritis

fibrous tumor
fibroma
neurofibroma
neuroma

filth eating
rhypophagy
scatophagy
eating of excrement

fingers abnormally long
arachnodactyly
dolichostenomelia

fingers/toes adhesion
ankylodactylia

finger communication
cheirology
chirology
dactylology

finger contracton
dactylospasm

fingers/toes defective
perodactylia
perodactyly

fingers/toes defective (cont.)
perodactylus
   individual involved

fingers of equal length
isodactylism

fingers in excess
hyperdactylia
hyperdactylism
hyperdactyly
polydactylism
polydactyly
   congenital development of supernumerary digits

fingers fused
syndactylia
syndactyly
syndactylous
zygodactyly

fingers inflamed
dactylitis

finger/toe lacking
adactyly
ectrodactylia
ectrodactylism
ectrodactyly
monodactylism
monodactyly
oligodactylia
oligodactyly
   congenital absence of one or more digits

finger largeness
dactylomegaly
macrodactylia
macrodactyly
macrodactylism
megadactyly
megalodactyly
   enlargement of one or more digits

finger shortness
brachydactylia
brachydactyly

finger slenderness
leptodactylous

finger/toe smallness
microdactylia
microdactylous
microdactyly
   smallness or shortness of the fingers or
   toes

finger thickness
pachydactylia
pachydactylous
pachydactyly

fingers unequal
anisodactylous
anisodactyly

fingerprint study
dactylography
dactyloscopy

first milk
colostrum
protogala
   first milk secreted at the termination of
   pregnancy

fish oils
eicosapentaenoic acids
omega-3 fatty acids

fish poisoning
ichthyismus
ichthyism

fish study
ichthyology

fishskin disease
ichthyosis
   thick, scaly skin

fission reproduction
schizogenesis

fissure in abdomen
celoschisis
celosomia
celosomus
kelosomus
   individual involved

fissure of sternum
sternoschisis

fistula operation
fistulectomy
fistuloenterostomy
fistulotomy

five children
quintipara
woman who has given birth
quintuplet
one of the children born

five day recurring
quintan
refers to symptom or disease

five fingered/toed
pentadactyl
pentadactyle

flame imagination
pyroptothymia
belief of engulfment in flames

flask shaped
lageniform

flat celled
planocellular

flat skull
platycephalic
platycephalous
platycephaly
platycrania
tapinocephalic
tapinocephaly
having a low, flat shape to the head

flatfootedness
pes planus

flatulence reliever
carminative agent

flea killer
pulicide

fleeing urge
poriomania

flesh eater
anthropophagy

flesh forming
sarcotic

fleshy tumor
sarcoma
malignant tumor of the connective tissue

floating kidney
nephroptosis

floating ribs
costae fluctuantes
costae fluitantes

flora and fauna
biota
collectively of a given region

flow of watery fluid
hydrorrhea

fluid accumulation
anasarca
in subcutaneous connective tissue
ascites
in abdomen
dropsy
old term for edema
edema
in tissues
hydrops
in any body tissues or cavities
hydrops fetalis
in the newborn

fluid in cranial vault
hydrocephalis
accompanied by enlargement of the
head and atrophy of the brain

fluid gravity measurer
pyknometer

fluid in joints
hydrarthrosis

fluid, watery
serum

fluidless
aneroid
anhydrous

fly killer
  muscicide

food
  aliment
  nutriment

food aversion
  anorexia nervosa
  sitophobia

food craving
  bulemia
  cissa
  citta
  cittosis
  phagomania
  pica
  sitiomania
  sitomania
    abnormal appetite and/or for abnormal
    substances

food inadequate
  hypoalimentation

food stagnation
  ischochymia
    in stomach

foot burning
  erythromelalgia

foot care
  pedicure

foot doctor
  chiropodist
  podiatrist
  podologist

foot gout
  podagra

foot-joint inflammation
  podarthritis

foot lacking
  sympus monopus
    congenital defect

foot largeness
  macropodia
  pes gigas

foot odor
  podobromhidrosis

foot operation
  tarsectomy
  tarsotomy

foot pain
  podalgia
  pododynia
  tarsalgia

foot smallness
  micropodia
  micropus
    individual involved

foot sole
  planta pedis

foot sole application
  suppedania
  suppedanum

foot thickness
  pachypodous

foot treatment
  chiropody

footless
  apodia
  apody
  monopus
  sirenomelia
  sirenomelus
    congenital absence

footless/headless
  acephalopodia
  acephalopodius

footprint
  ichnogram

forearm
  antebrachial
  antebrachium

forearm inner bone
  ulna

forearm shortness
  brachykerkic

64

foreign body extractor
protractor

foreign substance in blood
embolemia

foreign substance use
ergogenic

foremilk
colostrum

foreskin
prepuce
free fold of skin that covers the glans penis

foreskin lacking
aposthia

foreskin tightness
phimosis
narrowness of the opening of the prepuce

form equal
homeomorphous

formation of gas
aerogenesis
aerogenic
aerogenous
production and/or formation of gas

foul breath
halitosis
ozostomia

four arms
tetrabrachius

four breasts
tetramastia

four children
quadripara
woman who has given birth
quadruplet
one of the children born

four digits
tetradactyl

four ears
tetrotus

four extremity paralysis
quadriplegia

four eyelash rows
tetrastichiasis

four feet
tetrapus
congenital deformity

four-footed animal
quadruped

four hands
tetrachirus

four legs/arms
tetramelus
tetrascelus

fracture intentional
diaclasia
diclasis
osteoclasis

freak of nature
lusus naturae
extensive fetal malformation

freckle
ephelis
ephelides

freezing point finder
cryoscope

frenum operation
frenectomy
frenoplasty
frenotomy

frequent urination
micturitition
nocturia
nycturia
abnormally frequent urge to urinate

front and below
anteroinferior

front and side
anterolateral

front to back
anteroposterior

frontal headache
metopodynia

frost itch
pruritus hiemalis

fructose in blood
fructosemia
levulosemia

fructose in urine
fructosuria
levulosuria
excretion of fruit sugar in the urine

fruit sugar
levulose

function in excess
hyperfunction

function reduced
hypofunction

fundus viewer
funduscope
instrument to view the fundus of the eye

fungus suppressor
antimycotic

fungus disease
actinomycosis
mycosis
tinea
of the hair, skin or nails

fungus study
mycology

funnel chest
pectus excavatum

funnel-shaped
infundibular

fused ears
cyclotus
synotia
synotus

fuzz
pappus
first downy growth of beard

gait acceleration
festination
as seen in nervous disorders

gallbladder dilatation/distention
cholecystectasia

gallbladder inflammation
cholecystitis
pericholangitis
tissues around the bile duct
periangiocholitis
pericholecystitis
tissues around the gallbladder

gallbladder pain
cholecystalgia

gallbladder/intestine suture
cholecystenterorrhaphy

gallbladder operation
cholecystectomy
cholecystotomy
cholecystopexy
cholecystorrhaphy
cholecystenterostomy
cholecystocolostomy
cholecystoduodenostomy
cholecystostomy
cholecystogastrostomy
cholecystojejunostomy
choledochectomy
choledochostomy
choledochoplasty
choledochorrhaphy

gallbladder stones
cholecystolithiasis
cholelith
cholelithiasis
presence or formation of gallstones

gallbladder x-ray
cholecystogram
cholecystography

gallstone crushing
choledocholithotripsy
cholelithotripsy

ganglion inflammation
ganglionitis
periganglitis

gas/air in chest
pneumothorax
air or gas with fluid in the chest cavity

gas/air in intestines
aerenterectasia
meteorism
tympanites

gas/air in mediastinum
· *pneumomediastinum*

gas/air in peritoneal cavity
aeroperitonia
aeroperitoneum
pneumoperitoneum

gas/air vaginal distention
aerocolpos

gas/fluid removal
aspiration
suction to remove accumulation from a body cavity

gas in body tissues
aerosis

gas density measurer
aerometer

gas formation
aerogenesis
aerogenic
aerogenous

gas/liquid in tissues
hydropneumatosis

gas pain
tympanism
tympanites

gas pain (cont.)
distention due to air or gas in the intestine or peritoneal cavity

gas pressure measurer
manometer

gas in urine
pneumaturia

gas volume gauge
eudiometer
instrument to measure volume

gastric juice hormone
gastrin

gastric secretion lacking
achylia

genetic engineering
biotechnology
recombinant DNA

genital plastic operation
gynoplastics
reconstructive surgery of the female reproductive organs

genitals defective
agenosomia

geographic tongue
erythema migrans linguas
tongue with bare patches and thickened outer covering

germ absorbing
fomes
fomite
inanimate object that may retain infectious germs

germ cell
gonocyte

germ free
gnotobiota
gnotobiote
organisms without any contam-inating microorganisms

German measles
rubella

gestures/signs lacking

animia
loss of ability to communicate by means of gestures or signs

ataxic animia
inability to gesture due to paralysis or physical disorder

ghost hallucination

phantasmoscopia
phantasmoscopy

gigantism

somatomegaly

girdle pain

zonesthesia
sensation of tightness in lower abdominal area

gland/adenoids knife

adenotome
instrument to incise a gland or to remove adenoids

gland deficiency

adenasthenia

gland development

adenogenesis

gland disease

adenosis

gland enlargement

adenia

gland fibroid degeneration

adenofibrosis

gland hardening

adenosclerosis

gland hyperplasia

adenomatous

gland inflammation

adenitis
gland or lymph node
adenophlegmon
gland and connecting tissue
bartholinitis
major vestibular glands

gland inflammation (cont.)

myxadenitis
mucous gland
paradenitis
periadenitis
tissues surrounding a gland
perithyroiditis
thyroid gland capsules
thyroadenitis
thyroiditis
thyroid gland
strumitis
goiterous thyroid gland
sialadenitis
sialoadenitis
salivary gland
skeneitis
skenitis
glands near the urethra
sublinguitis
gland under the tongue
submaxillaritis
submaxillary gland
tarsadenitis
tarsal gland and plate

gland operation

adenectomy
adenotomy
parathyroidectomy
parotidectomy
pinealectomy
prostatectomy
prostatotomy
prostatolithotomy
sialoadenectomy
sialoadenotomy
sialolithotomy
sialodochoplasty
suprarenalectomy
thyroidectomy
thyroidotomy

gland/organ cells

parenchyma
distinguishing cells of a gland or organ

gland pain

adenalgia

gland softness

adenomalacia

gland stone
sebolith
in a sebaceous gland

gland tissue growth
adenomatosis

gland tumor
adenocarcinoma
adenocystoma
adenoepithelioma
adenolipoma
adenolymphoma
adenoma
adenosarcoma

gland in wrong place
adenectopia
malposition or displacement of a gland

glandlike
adeniform
adenoid
adenose
adenous

glass tube
buret
burette
pipet
pipette
graduated tube used to deliver a measured amount of liquid or gas

glasslike
hyaline
hyaloid
vitreous

glaucoma operation
sclerostomy

globular tumor
spheroma

globulin in urine
globulinuria

glucose in blood
glycemia

god of medicine
Aesculapius
Asklepios
Greek god of medicine

goiter
thyrocele
chronic enlargement of the thyroid gland

goiter inflammation
strumitis

goiter operation
strumectomy

gold therapy
chrysotherapy
treatment of disease by the administration of gold salts

gonococci in blood
gonococcemia

gout in foot
podagra
especially of the great toe

gout in knee joint
gonagra

gout in neck
trachelagra

gout reliever
antarthritic
antiarthritic
uricosuric

gouty deposit in joint
arthrolith
tophus
chalkstone*
*obsolete term

grafting
heteroosteoplasty
heteroplasty
grafting a bone taken from an animal
heterotransplantation
grafting any part taken from a different species
homograft
homoplasty
homotransplantation
grafting taken from same species

gravel in urine
uropsammus

gray matter inflammation
poliomyelitis
of the spinal cord

grayness of hair
   canities
   poliosis

greasy
   oleaginous

greatness delusion
   megalomania
   megalomaniac

green sickness
   chlorosis
   chlorotic
     anemic disease in young females

green vision
   chloropsia

groin area
   inguinal

groin pain
   inguinodynia

groove between nates
   gluteal furrow
   sulcus gluteus

groove on brain
   sulcus
     a depression on the brain surface separating the folds

growth
   accretion

gum
   gingiva
     pertaining to area of the mouth

gum abscess
   gumboil
   parulis

gum bleeding
   ulorrhagia

gum inflammation
   gingivitis
   gingivoglossitis
     gums and tongue
   gingivostomatitis
     gums and mouth

gum operation
   gingivectomy
   ulotomy

H

hair beading
   monilethrix
   moniliform
     hereditary condition of marked constrictions in the hair

hair brittleness
   sclerothrix
   trichatrophia
   trichorrhexis

hair calcified
   tricholith

hair component
   keratin
     principal component of hair

hair deficiency
   hypotrichiasis
   hypotrichosis
   oligotrichia
   oligotrichosis

hair disease
   trichitis
   trichomycosis
   trichopathy

hair in excess
   hypertrichosis
   polytrichia
     excessive growth of hair over all or part of the body

hair follicles inflamed
   acne decalvans
   folliculitis
   perifolliculitis

hair fungus disease
trichomycosis
trichosporosis

hair gray
canities
poliosis

hair growth abnormal
hirsutism
paratrichosis
pilosis
hypertrichosis lanuginosa
on the body of the fetus

hair harsh/dry
sclerothrix
sclerotrichia
xerasia

hair inversion
trichiasis
turning inward of the hair surrounding an opening

hair loss
acomia
for any reason
alopecia
total or partial loss
alopecia aereata
in patches
alopecia cicatrisata
in circular patches due to atrophy of the skin
alopecia senilis
due to aging
alopecia symptomatica
due to systemic or psychogenic causes
alopecia totalis
alopecia universalis
all over the body
atrichia
may be congenital or acquired
madarosis
trichosis
loss of eyelashes/eyebrows
oligotrichia
scarcity of hair

hair loss (cont.)
ophiasis
a serpentine form of baldness
phalacrosis
obsolete term for baldness
psilosis
due to a cutaneous disorder

hair of lower abdomen
pubescence
hair that grows at puberty

hair in nose
vibrissa

hair plucking
trichologia
trichology
the science of hair
trichotillomania
uncontrollable desire to pull out hair

hair removing
decalvent
depilate
depilation
depilatory
epilate
epilation
epilatory

hair scarcity
oligotrichia

hair-shaped
filiform

hair smooth/straight
leiotrichous

hair splitting
distrix
schizotrichia

hair-touch sensation
trichoesthesia
experienced when a hair is touched
trichoesthesiometer
instrument to measure the sensation

hair whiteness
leukotrichia
leukotrichous

hairless
> *glabrous*
>> smooth and bare

hairlike
> *trichoid*

hairy
> *hirsute*
> *hirsutism*
> *pilar*
> *pilary*
> *pilose*

hairy tongue
> *glossotrichia*
> *trichoglossia*
> *nigrities linguae*
>> black hairy tongue

hallucinatory condition
> *hallucinosis*

hammer bone of ear
> *malleus*

hammer nose
> *rhinophyma*

hand
> *manus*

hand arthritis
> *chirarthritis*

hand burning
> *erythromelalgia*
>> abnormal burning sensation of hands or feet

hand dexterity
> *ambidexter*
> *ambidextrous*
>> individual that uses either hand equally well

hand excessive number
> *polycheiria*
> *polychiria*

hand joint
> *articulatio manus*

hand joint contraction
> *acrocontracture*
>> shortening of the muscles in the joints of hands or feet

hand joint inflammation
> *chirarthritis*

hand lacking
> *acheiria*
> *achiria*
>> also sense of loss

hand largeness
> *acrodolichomelia*
> *cheiromegaly*
> *chiromegaly*
> *megalocheiria*

hand operation
> *cheiroplasty*
> *chiroplasty*

hand smallness
> *microcheiria*
> *microchiria*

hand spasm
> *acromyotonia*
> *acromyotonus*

hand sweat increased
> *acrohyperhidrosis*

hand underdeveloped
> *perochirus*
>> individual with congenital defect

handless/headless
> *acephalocheirus*
> *acephalochirus*
>> malformed fetus without hands or head

handwriting study
> *graphology*

hanging breast operation
> *mammoplasty*
> *mastopexy*
> *mazopexy*

hard palate
> *palatum durum*
>> roof of the mouth

hardening
sclerema
scleroma
sclerosis

hardening of bone
osteosclerosis

hardness measurer
sclerometer

hardness of an organ
scirrhosity

hare's eye
lagophthalmic
lagophthalmos
inability to close the eye

harelip
chiloschisis
cleft lip
congenital opening

harmful
deleteriour
noxious
toxin

harmless
innocuous
innoxious

hatred for children
misopedia
misopedy

hatred for mankind
misanthropy
aversion to people

hatred for marriage
misogamy

hatred for newness
misoneism

hatred for women
misogyny

hay fever
pollenosis
pollinosis
allergic reaction to pollen

head lacking
deranencephalia
deranencephaly

head cold
coryza
acute rhinitis

head largeness
macrocephalia
macrocephaly
megalocephaly

head measurer
cephalometer

head narrowness
stenocephalia
stenocephalic
stenocephalous
stenocephaly

head/neck lacking
atrachelocephalus
fetus with head and neck either lacking
or undeveloped

head pointed
acrocephalia
acrocephalic
acrocephaly
oxycephalic
oxycephaly
turricephaly

head smallness
microcephalia
microcephalism
microcephaly
microcephalus
nanocephalous
nanocaphaly

head to tail
cephalocaudal

head/thorax
cephalothoracic

head-top concave
clinocephaly

headache
cephalalgia
encephalalgia
general term
metopodynia
frontal headache
migraine
vascular cause
psychalalgia
psychalgia
psychalgic
usually caused by depression

headless
acephalus
acephalous

head/arm lacking
abrachiocephalus
abrachiocephaly
acephalobrachius
born without head and arms

head/foot lacking
acephalopodia
acephalopodius
born without head and feet

head/hand lacking
acephalocheirus
acephalochirus
born without head and hands

head/heart lacking
acephalocardia
born without head and heart

head/mouth lacking
acephalostomia
having a mouthlike opening in the upper
part of neck/chest

head/spine lacking
acephalorrhachia
born without head and spinal column

head/thorax lacking
acephalothorus
born without head and chest

healing by massage
naprapathy

health anxiety
hypochondriac
hypochondriasis

healthy old age
agerasia

hearing acuteness
hyperacusia
hyperacusis
exceptionally acute sense of hearing

hearing dysfunction
diplacusis

hearing measurer
audiometer
audiometry

heart abnormally situated
bathycardia
ectocardia
exocardia

heart with air
aerendocardia

heart arrest
cardioplegic solution
induced condition

heart assist
counterpulsation
technique for decreasing workload of
the heart by using an external pump

heart beat irregular
arrhythmia
cardiataxia
dysrhythmia
tumultus cordis

heart beat rapid
tachycardia

heart beat slow
brachycardia
bradycardia

heart chamber with air/gas
pneumatocardia

heart development
cardiogenesis

heart dilatation
cardiectasis

heart disease
cardiomyopathy
cardiopathy
    designating primarily heart muscle disease

heart disease treatment
cardiotherapy

heart displacement
ectocardia
exocardia
cardioptosia
cardioptosis

heart enlargement
auxocardia
bucardia
cardiomegaly
cor bovinum
macrocardius

heart/great vessels
angiocardiopathy

heart hernia
cardiocele
    protrusion of the heart through a wound or opening of the diphragm

heart inflammation
carditis
cardiopericarditis
endocarditis

heart lacking
acardia
acardiac
acardiacus
    born without heart

heart largeness
cardiomegaly
macrocardia
macrocardius
megalocardia

heart membrane
endocardium
    lines the inner cavities of the heart

heart membrane (cont.)
pericardium
    surrounds the heart

heart monitor
cardiography
    graphic recording of a physical or functional aspect of the heart

heart operation
cardiectomy
cardiocentesis
cardio-omentopexy
cardiopericardiopexy
cardiopuncture
cardiorrhaphy
cardiomyopexy
cardioplasty
cardiotomy

heart pain
cardialgia
cardiodynia

heart paralysis
cardioplegia
    use of chemicals or cold to stop contractions during surgery

heart puncture
cardiocentesis
cardiopuncture

heart on right side
dextrocardia

heart rupture
cardiorrhexis

heart-shaped
cordate
cordiform

heart smallness
microcardia
microcardius

heart softness
cardiomalacia
    softening of the muscular substances of the heart

heart stimulant
digitalis
dobutamine
ouabain
strophanthin

heart stroke
angina pectoris

heart study
cardiology

heart suture
cardiorrhaphy

heartburn
pyrosis

heart/head missing
acephalocardius
born without head and heart

heat deprivation
thermosteresis

heat insensibility
thermanalgesia
thermoanalgesia
thermoanesthesia

heat loss
thermolytic
thermolysis
dissipation of bodily heat such as by
evaporation

heat pain
thermalgesia
thermoalgesia

heat-producing
calorifacient

heat production measurer
calorimeter

heat sensitiveness
thermesthesia
thermoesthesia

heating tissues
diathermy
to decrease resistance to passage of radiation, electrical current or ultrasound

heel bone
calcaneus

heel pain
calcaneodynia

hemoglobin deficiency
oligochromemia
insufficient amount of hemoglobin in all
the red blood cells

hemoglobin excess
hemoglobinemia
excessive amount in the blood

hemoglobin measurer
hemoglobinometer

hemoglobin separation
hemolysis

hemoglobin in urine
hemoglobinuria

hemolysis preventer
antihemolytic

hemorrhage control
electrohemostasis

hemorrhage from ear
otorrhagia

hemorrhage from eye
ophthalmorrhagia

hemorrhage of intestine
enterorrhagia

hemorrhage of kidney
nephrorrhagia

hemorrhage of penis
balanorrhagia
inflammation with discharge of pus

hemorrhage of spinal cord
hematomyelia
hemorrhage into the substance of the
spinal cord

hemorrhage of stomach
gastrorrhagia

hemorrhage of veins
phleborrhagia

hemp poisoning
cannabism

heparin in blood
heparinemia

hernia of brain
cephalocele
encephalocele

hernia of choroid
choriocele
  coat of the eye

hernia of diaphragm
diaphragmatocele

hernia with fatty tissue
adipocele
lipocele
  hernia containing fat

hernia knife
herniotome
  surgical instrument

hernia with omentum
epiplocele
epiploenterocele

hernia repair
hernioplasty
herniorrhaphy
herniotomy

hernia of spleen
lienocele

hernia of testes
orchiocele

hernia of umbilicus
omphalocele
  protrusion at birth of part of the intestine
  through the abdominal wall

hernia of vagina
colpocele
vaginocele

heroin
diacetylmorphine

hinge joint
ginglymus

hip bone/socket
os coxae

hip joint
articulatio coxae

hip joint disease
coxarthropathy

hip operation
hemipelvectomy

hip pain
coxalgia
coxodynia

hippuric acid in urine
hippuria
  excessive amounts

histamine in blood
histidemia
  also reflected in excess urine levels

histidine in urine
histidinuria
  also reflected in excess blood levels

histone in urine
histonuria

hives
urticaria

home life aversion
apodemialgia

homogentisic acid in urine
alkaptonuria

homosexuality
lesbianism
sapphism
  among females

hook shaped
unciform
uncinate

hookworm disease
ancylostomiasis
necatoriasis
  infestation with hookworms

hops
humulus

hops bitter
humulin
lupulin

hormone production
hormonopoiesis

horn component
keratin

horny
keratic
keratinous

horny skin
keratosis
any horny growth(e.g., wart or callus)

horse bone inflammation
peditis

hospital-related
nosocomial

housefly
musca domestica

hoy
phencyclidine (PCP)

human in form
anthropomorphism

humpbacked deformity
gibbosity
kyphosis

hunger in excess
bulimia
resulting from a mental disorder

hyalin in urine
hyalinuria

hydrochloric acid excess
hyperchlorhydria
in the gastric juice

hydrochloric acid low
hypochlorhydria

hydrogen sulfide in blood
hydrothionemia

hydrogen sulfide in urine
hydrothionuria

hydrolysis of proteins
proteolysis
splitting of proteins

hymen inflammation
hymenitis

hymen operation
hymenectomy
hymenotomy

hymen suture
hymenorrhaphy

hypnosis
autohypnosis
autohypnotic
induced by oneself
heterohypnosis
induced by another

hysteria controller
hysterofrenic

hysterical laughter
cachinnation

hysterical paralysis
pseudoplegia

I

idiocy
anoesia
anoia
inability to understand

idiopathic vomiting
autemesia

ileum inflammation
ileitis
ileocolitis
ileum and colon

ileum operation
  ileectomy
  ileotomy
  ileocecostomy
  ileocolostomy
  ileoileostomy
  ileosigmoidostomy
  ileostomy

ileum suture
  ileorrhaphy

ill health
  cachectic
  cachexia

illuminated viewer
  caveascope
  cavernoscope
  celoscope
    instrument for examining the interior of a
    body cavity

image perception in excess
  polyopia
  polyopsia
    seeing more than one image

imaginary odors
  cacosmia
  parosmia

immunity study
  immunology

impairment of senses
  dysesthesia
    of any sense, especially sense of touch

imperforate cardiac opening
  atretogastria

imperforate opening
  atresic
  atresia
  atretic

imperforate pupil
  atresia iridis
  atretopsia

imperforate pyloric orifice
  atretogastria

imperforate urethra
  atreturethria

imperforate urinary bladder
  atretocystia

impervious to heat
  adiathermancy

impregnated ovum
  cytula

inability to copy writing
  dysantigraphia

inability to decide
  abulia
  abulic
    deficiency of will power, initiative or
    drive

inability to fix attention
  aprosexia

inability to form sentences
  acataphasia

inability to locate sensation
  atopognosia
  atopognosis

inability for mathematics
  acalculia
    inability to calculate

inability to name objects
  anomia
  nominal aphasia

inability to recognize by touch
  astereognosis
  tactile amnesia
  stereoagnosis
  stereoanesthesia

inability to relax
  achalasia
    specifically the hollow muscular organs

inability to arise
  ananastasia
    from a sitting position

inability to sit
  acathisia

inability to sit (cont.)
akathisia
akatizia
    motor restlessness, muscle quivering

inability to sleep
agrypnia
insomnia

inability to speak
aphasia

inability to stand
astasic
astatic
    to maintain an erect position
astasia abasia
    to stand or walk

inability to swallow
aphagia

inability to urinate
anuria
anuric

inability to write
agraphia
    loss of ability to write
agraphic
anorthography
    loss of ability to write correctly

inactive
quiescent

incoherence of speech
allophasis

incontinence of urine
enuresis
enuretic
uracrasia

incus operation
incudectomy
    of the ear

indican in urine
indicanuria

indifferent
adiphoria
    failure to respond to stimuli

indifferent (cont.)
pseudodementia
    exaggerated indifference to one's sur-
    roundings

indigestion
dyspepsia
dyspeptic

indigo in urine
indigouria
indiguria

indole in urine
indoluria

indolacetic acid in urine
indolaceturia

indoxyl in urine
indoxyluria
    secreted as indican

infant cry
vagitus

infantile paralysis
poliomyelitis

inferiority conscious
micromania

inflamed adnexa uteri
adnexitis
annexitis
    including the tubes, ligaments, ovaries

inflamed amnion
amnionitis

inflamed aorta
aortitis

inflamed appendix
appendicitis

inflamed artery
arteritis

inflamed bone
osteitis
ostitis
myelitis
    spinal cord or bone marrow

inflamed bone (cont.)
  osteomyelitis
    marrow, bone and cartilage
  periostitis
    connective tissue

inflamed brain
  cerebritis
  encephalitis
  meningoencephalitis

inflamed breast
  mastitis

inflamed bronchial glands
  bronchoadenitis

inflamed cheek
  melitis

inflamed ear
  otitis
  panotitis

inflamed eye
  blepharitis
    eyelid
  choroiditis
    choroid
  ophthalmia
  ophthalmitis
    eye and conjunctiva
  panophthalmia
  panophthalmitis
    entire eyeball structure
  scleritis
  sclerotitis
    eyeball coating
  trachoma
    granular conjunctivitis

inflamed Fallopian tube
  salpingitis
  syringitis
    also of Eustachian tube

inflamed finger
  dactylitis

inflamed foreskin
  phimosis
  phimotic

inflamed glands
  adenitis

inflamed gums
  gingivitis

inflamed hair follicles
  sycosis

inflamed intestines
  enteritis
    any part of the intestinal tract
  cecitis
  typhlitis
    cecum
  colitis
    colon
  enterocolitis
    small intestine and colon
  enterogastritis
  gastroenteritis
    intestine and stomach
  ileitis
    ileum
  ileocolitis
    ileum and colon
  mucoenteritis
    mucous membrane of intestine
  paratyphlitis
    connective tissue near cecum
  pericecitis
    cecum serosa
  perienteritis
    intestinal peritoneum
  perijejunitis
    tissues around the jejunum
  proctitis
    rectum or anus
  rectocolitis
    rectum and colon
  seroenteritis
    small intestine serous covering
  sigmoiditis

inflamed joint
  arthritis
  periarthritis
    around the joint
  polyarthritis
    several joints

inflamed joint membrane
synovitis

inflamed kidney
nephritis
pyelitis
   pelvis of a kidney
pyelonephritis
   kidney and its pelvis
pyonephritis
   with pus formation

inflamed larynx
laryngitis
laryngopharyngitis
   larynx and pharynx
laryngotracheitis
   larynx and trachea
laryngotracheobronchitis
   larynx, trachea and bronchi

inflamed ligament
syndesmitis

inflamed liver
hepatitis

inflamed lungs
baritosis
   due to barium inhalation
kaolinosis
   from inhaling kaolin dust
pneumoenteritis
   lungs and intestine
pneumonia
pneumonitis
pulmonitis
   of the lungs proper

inflamed marrow/bone
osteomyelitis

inflamed mouth
stomatitis

inflamed mucous gland
myxadenitis

inflamed nail
onychia
onyxitis
   nail matrix

inflamed nail (cont.)
paronychia
whitlow
   with pus formation

inflamed nerve
neuritis
mononeuritis
   a single nerve
neurochorioretinitis
neurochoroiditis
neuroretinitis
   retinal nerves
neuromyelitis
   nerves and spinal cord
neuromyositis
   nerves and muscles
perineuritis
   the perineurial sheath enclosing a bundle of nerves

inflamed nipple
mammillitis

inflamed nostril
rhinitis
   mucous membranes
rhinoantritis
   mucous membrane and sinus
rhinolaryngitis
   mucous membrane and larynx
rhinopharyngitis
   nose and pharynx

inflamed nympha
nymphitis
   minor lips

inflamed ovaries
oophoritis
ovaritis
oophorosalpingitis
ovariosalpingitis
   ovary and oviduct

inflamed palate
palatitis

inflamed pancreas
pancreatitis

82

inflamed parotid gland
parotitis
the mumps

inflamed pericardium
pericarditis

inflamed periosteum
periostitis
membrane covering bones

inflamed peritoneum
peritonitis
membrane covering abdominal organs

inflamed pharynx
pharyngitis
pharyngolaryngitis
pharynx and larynx
pharyngorhinitis
with rhinitis
pharyngotonsillitis
with tonsillitis

inflamed pleura
pleurisy
pleuritis
pleurohepatitis
pleura and liver
pleuropericarditis
with pericarditis

inflamed prepuce
acroposthitis
posthitis

inflamed rectum
proctitis

inflamed retina
retinitis
retinochoroiditis
retina and choroid
retinopapillitis
retina and optic disk

inflamed skin
dermatitis
acrodermatitis
of an extremity
prurigo
itching and inflammation of the papules

inflamed skin (cont.)
pyoderma
pyodermatitis
with pus
radiodermatitis
caused by radioactivity
toxicodermatitis
caused by poison

inflamed spinal cord
myelitis
meningomyelitis
spinal cord and its membranes
poliomyelitis
gray matter
radiculitis
spinal nerve root
syringomyelitis
with syringomyelia

inflamed spleen
splenitis
perisplenitis
membrane covering the spleen

inflamed stomach
gastritis
enterogastritis
gastroenteritis
stomach and intestine
gastroesophagitis
stomach and esophagus
gastroduodenitis
stomach and duodenum
perigastritis
stomach serosa
pyloritis
pylorus

inflamed subcutaneous fatty tissue
adipositis
panniculitis

inflamed synovial membrane
synovitis

inflamed tendon
tendinitis
tendonitis
tenonitis
tenositis

inflamed testicles
  orchitis

inflamed thyroid
  thyroiditis

inflamed tongue
  glossitis
  subglossitis
  sublinguitis

inflamed tonsil
  tonsillitis
  adenopharyngitis
  pharyngotonsillitis
    tonsils and pharynx

inflamed trachea
  tracheitis
  trachitis
  tracheobronchitis
    trachea and bronchi
  tracheopyosis
    purulent inflammation

inflamed ureter
  ureteritis
  ureteropyelitis
    ureter and kidney pelvis
  ureteropyelonephritis
    ureter, kidney and pelvis
  ureteropyosis
    with purulent exudation

inflamed urethra
  urethritis
  urethrocystis
  urethrotrigonitis
    urethra and bladder

inflamed uterus
  metritis
  uteritis
  metrolymphangitis
    lymphatic vessels
  metroperitonitis
    uterus and peritoneum
  metrophlebitis
    veins of the uterus
  metrosalpingitis
    uterus and oviducts

inflamed uvea
  uveitis

inflamed uvula
  staphylitis
  uvulitis

inflamed vein
  phlebitis
  mesophlebitis
    middle coat of the vein
  periangitis
    outside tissues

inflamed vertebra
  spondylitis
  perispondylitis
    tissues around the vertebrae
  spondylopyosis
    accompanied by pus

inflamed vessel
  angiitis
  angitis
  angiodermatitis
    skin vessels
  angiotitis
    ear blood vessels

inflamed windpipe
  tracheitis
  trachitis

inflammation reliever
  antiphlogistic
  antipyrotic

inflatable cervix dilator
  hystereurynter
    instrument for dilating the uterus

ingrowing nail
  unguis incarnatus

inguinal pain
  bubonalgia
  inguinodynia

inhale/exhale measurer
  spirometer

injury
  trauma

inosital in blood
inosemia
excess of fibrin in the blood

inosital in urine
inosituria
inosuria

insanity over religion
hieromania

insensibility to pain
analgesia

insomnia
agrypnia
ahypnia
ahypnosis

insulin in blood
insulinemia
excessive amounts

insulin diminishing
insulinopenic

insulin formation
insulinogenesis

insulin tumor
insulinoma
tumor of the beta cells of the islets of Langerhans

intellectual alertness
prothymia

intellectual loss
dementia

interbreeding
amphimixis

intercourse
coitus
copulation
pareunia

intercourse with animals
zooerastia

intercourse painful
dyspareunia

internal hernia
entocele

internal origin
autopathic
autopathy
disease without apparent external cause

internal secretion glands
endocrine glands

internal secretion study
endocrinology

interstitial pregnancy
salpingysterocyesis

intestinal
enteric
enteral

intestinal bloody discharge
hematorrhea

intestinal contraction/motion
peristalsis

intestinal "crawling"
diastalsis
type of downward moving wave in small intestine during the digestive process

intestinal crusher
splanchnotribe
instrument for crushing a segment of the intestine

intestinal dilatation
enterectasis

intestinal disease
enteromycosis
fungal disease
enteropathy
any intestinal disease

intestinal gas/air
aerenterectasia
meteorism
tympanites

intestinal hemorrhage
enterorrhagia
enterostaxis

intestinal hernia

enterocele
hernia containing a loop of intestine
enteroepiplocele
hernia of the omentum
enterocystocele
involving intestine and bladder

intestinal inflammation

cecitis
typhlitis
typhlenteritis
of the cecum
diverticulitis
of intestinal sacs
enteritis
in general
enterocolitis
small intestine and colon
enterogastritis
gastroenteritis
intestine and stomach
mucoenteritis
of the mucous membrane
paratyphlitis
of the connective tissue near the cecum
periappendicitis
of tissues around the appendix
pericecitis
of the cecum serosa
perienteritis
of the intestinal peritoneum
perijejunitis
of the tissue around the jejunum
perityphlitis
obsolete term for periappendicitis
seroenteritis
small intestine serous covering
typhlodicliditis
of the ileocecal valve

intestinal irritation

clyster
enema

intestine lacking

anenterous

intestine largeness

enteromegalia

intestine largeness (cont.)

enteromegaly
megaloenteron

intestinal obstruction

splanchnemphraxis
in general
volvulus
twisting

intestinal operation

cecectomy
cecocolostomy
cecoileostomy
cecosigmoidostomy
cecostomy
cecotomy
celioenterotomy
typhlectomy
typhlostomy
typhlotomy
involving the cecum
colectomy
colocolostomy
colohepatopexy
coloproctostomy
colosigmoidostomy
colostomy
colotomy
diverticulectomy
enterectomy
enterocolectomy
enterocolostomy
enteroenterostomy
enteropexy
enteroplasty
enterostomy
enterotomy
involving the colon
ileectomy
ileocecostomy
ileocolostomy
ileoileostomy
ileosigmoidostomy
ileostomy
ileotomy
involving the ileum
laparoenterotomy
proctectomy

Intestinal operation (cont.)
proctopexy
proctoplasty
proctosigmoidectomy
proctostomy
proctotomy
rectectomy
rectopexy
rectosigmoidectomy
rectostomy
rectotomy
　involving the rectum
sigmoidectomy
sigmoidopexy
sigmoidoproctostomy
sigmoidorectostomy
sigmoidosigmoidostomy
sigmoidostomy
sigmoidotomy
　involving the sigmoid colon

intestine pain
enteralgia
enterodynia

intestinal paralysis
adynamic ileus
enteroplegia
paralytic ileus

intestinal peristalsis lacking
aperistalsis

intestinal prolapse
coloptosis
enteroptosis

intestinal puncture
enterocentesis
　surgical puncture

intestinal rumbling
barborygmus
rugitus

intestinal rupture
enterorrhexis

intestinal sac
diverticulum
　may be congenital or acquired

intestinal stone
enterolith

intestinal stricture
enterostenosis

intestinal suture
cecorrhaphy
enterorrhaphy

intestinal toxemia
scatemia
　blood poisoning

intestinal toxins
clostridium bacteria

intestinal viewer
enteroscope

intestine worm medicine
anthelmintic
santonin

involuntary urination
enuresis
nocturnal enuresis
nocturia
nycturia
　bedwetting, usually at night

Iodine sickness
iodism
iododerma

iris adhesion
synechia
　also applies to any adhesion

iris angle
angulus iridis

iris atrophy
iridoleptynsis

iris eversion
iridectropium

iris hemorrhage
iridemia

iris inflammation
iritis
choroidoiritis

iris inflammation (cont.)
iridochoroiditis
iris and choroid
iridocapsulitis
iris and capsule
iridocyclitis
iris and ciliary body
iridoperiphakitis
iris and part of capsule
scleroiritis
iris and sclera
sclerokeratoiritis
iris, sclera and cornea

iris inversion
iridentropium

iris knife
corectome
iridectome
instrument for iris removal

iris lacking
aniridia
irideremia
congenital absence

iris operation
iridoavulsion
iridectomy
iridotomy
iritomy
iritoectomy
iridocyclectomy
iridocystectomy
iridosclerotomy
sclerectoiridectomy

iris paralysis
iridoparalysis
iridoplegia

iris prolapse
iridoptosis
protrusion through a wound or ulcer

iris ring
annulus iridis

iris rupture
iridorrhexis

iris softness
iridomalacia

iris tremor
hippus
spasmodic, rhythmical dilation and constriction

iris thickening
iridauxesis

iron deficiency
sideropenia

iron worker disease
siderosis

isolation hospital
lazaret
lazaretto

itching
pruritus

itching reliever
antipruritic

itching skin
neurodermatitis

jargon
glossolalia
unintelligible jargon

jaundice
icteric
icterus

jaundice causing
icterogenic

jaw bone
mandible

jaws equal size
isognathous

jaw force measurer
  gnathodynamometer
    instrument that records the force exerted in closing jaws

jaw inflammation
  gnathitis
    also refers to inflammation of the cheek

jaw lacking
  agnathia
  agnathus
  agnathous

jaw largeness
  macrognathia
  macrognathic
  megagnathia

jaws mismatched
  anisognathous

jaw muscle
  masseter
    raises the lower jaw

jaw operation
  alveolectomy
  alveoloplasty
  alveoplasty
  alveolotomy
  gnathoplasty

jaw projecting
  hypognathia
  prognathism
  prognathic
  prognathous

jaw shortness
  brachygnathia

jaw smallness
  micrognathia

jejunum/ileum
  jejunoileal

jejunum inflammation
  jejunitis
  jejunoileitis
    jejunum and ileum

jejunum operation
  jejunectomy
  jejunocolostomy
  jejunoileostomy
  jejunojejunostomy
  jejunoplasty
  jejunostomy
  jejunotomy
  nestiostomy

joint with air
  pneumarthrosis
    presence of air in a joint

joint ball-and-socket
  enarthrosis

joint disease
  arthropathy
  osteoarthritis
  osteoarthrosis
    degenerative disease of the joints

joint drainage
  arthrocentesis
  arthrostomy

joint flexion measurer
  fleximeter
  goniometer

joint fusion
  arthrodesis
  symphysis
  synarthrosis

joint gouty deposit
  arthrolith
  tophus
  *chalkstone**
    *obsolete term

joints of hand contracted
  acrocontracture
    shortening of muscles in the joints of hands or feet

joint inflammation
  arthritic
  arthritis
  monarthric
  monarticular

joint inflammation (cont.)
monoarthritis
pertaining to a single joint
panarthritis
polyarthritis
of several joints
periarthritis
of tissues around a joint
synovitis
of the synovial membrane

joint lubricant
synovia
clear fluid that functions to lubricate a joint

joint mobility reduction
arthroereisis
arthrarisis

joint movement measurer
arthrometer
arthrometry
goniometer
measurement of the range of movement of a joint

joint operation
arthrectomy
arthrotomy
arthrolysis
arthroplasty
arthrostomy
synovectomy
villusectomy

joint pain
arthralgia
arthralgic
arthrodynia
arthrodynic
polyarthralgia

joint pus
pyarthrosis
suppurative arthritis

joint rigidity
acampsia

joint sensation
arthresthesia

joint stiffness
ankylosis
bony ankylosis
synostosis
true ankylosis

joint suppuration
arthroempyesis

joint viewer
arthroscope
arthroendoscopy
instrument to view inside joint
arthroscopy
examining the inside of a joint with an endoscope

jumbling words
paraphrasia

K

ketone bodies in blood
ketonemia

ketone bodies in urine
ketonuria
hyperketonuria

kidneys
nephric
nephroid
nephrons
renal
shape of a kidney

kidney abscess
nephrapostasis

kidney connective tissue
perinephrium
connective tissue and fat surrounding a kidney

kidney cyst
nephrocystosis

kidney dilatation
nephrectasis

kidney disease
nephrasthenia
nephronophthisis
nephropathy
nephrosis
renopathy

kidney displacement
nephrocele
nephrocelon
hernial displacement of a kidney

kidney function assessment
nephrogram
nephrography
nephrotomogram
nephrotomography
renogram
renography

kidney function lost/diminished
nephratonia
nephratony
renoprival

kidney floating
nephrospasia
nephrospasis
attachment of the organ only by the blood vessels

kidney hardness
nephrosclerosis
nephrosclerotic

kidney hemorrhage
nephremorrhagia
nephrorrhagia
hemorrhage from or into the kidney

kidney inflammation
glomerulonephritis
nephritis
nephrophthisis
nephritides
lithonephritis

kidney inflammation (cont.)
nephropyelitis
pyelitis
pyelonephritis
of the kidney pelvis
perinephritis
of tissues around a kidney
pyelocystitis
urinary bladder and the pelvis of a kidney
pyonephritis
accompanied by pus

kidney nourishment
nephrotrophic
nephrotropic
renotrophic
renotrophin
renotropin

kidney operation
nephrectomy
nephrotomy
nephrocapsectomy
nephrocystanastamosis
nephrolithotomy
nephropexy
nephropyeloplasty
nephrostomy
nephroureterectomy
pyelolithotomy
pyeloplasty
pyelostomy
pyelotomy

kidney origination
nephrogenetic
nephrogenic
nephrogenous
renogenic
giving rise to kidney tissue

kidney pain
nephralgia

kidney pelvis distention
hydropyonephrosis

kidney prolapse
nephroptosia
nephroptosis

kidney proximity
adrenal
located near or upon the kidney

kidney shaped
nephroid
reniform

kidney softening
nephromalacia

kidney stone
nephrolith
nephrocalcinosis
nephrolithiasis
pyonephrolithiasis
accompanied by pus

kidney suture
nephrorrhaphy

kidney study/treatment
nephrology

kidney toxin
nephrolysin
antibody that causes destruction of the cells of the kidneys
nephrotoxic
nephrotoxin
cytotoxin specific for cells of the kidney

kidney tumor
nephroadenoma
nephroblastema
nephroblastoma
nephroma
nephroncus

kidney ulceration
nephrelcosis

kidney vessels
glomerulus
renovascular

killing offspring
feticide
before birth
infanticide
after birth

knee inflammation
gonarthritis
gonitis
meniscitis
of the interarticular cartilage

knee-jerk
patellar reflex

knee joint
articulatio genus

knee joint inflammation
gonarthritis
gonarthromeningitis

knee joint operation
gonarthrotomy
incision into the knee joint

knee pain
gonalgia

knee tumor
gonatocele

kneecap
patella

knock-knee
genu valgum
tibia valga

L

labor difficult
dystocia

labor producer
oxytocic
parturifacient
an agent that produces or accelerates labor

labyrinth inflammation
labyrinthitis

labyrinth operation
labyrinthectomy
labyrinthotomy

lack of alkalinity
acidosis
insufficient amount of alkali/base in the blood

lack of bile pigment
acholuria
acholuric
in the urine

lack of bile secretion
acholia

lack of heart
acardia
acardius

lack of limbs
ectromelia

lack of mental ability
amentia
dementia

lack of nutrition
cachexia
general wasting seen during a chronic illness

lack of pigmentation
achromatosis

lack of pupil
acorea

lack of ribs
apleuria

lack of skin pigment
achromasia
achromia

lack of strength
hyposthenia

lack of teeth
adontia
adontism
edentate
edentulous

lack of teeth (cont.)
hypodontia
oligodontia

lack of testes
agenitalism
anorchia
anorchidism
anorchism
having no testes
monorchid
monorchidic
monorchidism
monorchis
monorchism
having only one testis

lack of trunk
acormus
fetus born without a torso

lacrimal duct stone
dacryolith
ophthalmolith
also called a tear stone

lacrimal gland pain
dacryoadenalgia

lacrimal sac protrusion
dacryocele
dacryocystocele

lactation diminisher
antigalactagogue
antigalactic
diminishing or suppressing the secretion of milk

lactic acid in blood
lactacidemia
lacticacidemia

lactiferous duct inflamed
galactophoritis

lactose in urine
lactosuria

lamina operation
laminectomy
hemilaminectomy
rachiotomy

lamina operation (cont.)
rachitomy
spondylotomy

languor of organs
atonia
atonicity
atony
weakness of any organ, especially the muscles

lanolin
adeps lanae hydrosus
wool fat (anhydrous)

large-footed
pachypodous

large hands
cheiromegaly
chiromegaly
megalocheiric
megalochiria

large head
macrocephalia
macrocephaly
macrocephalous
macrocephalus
megacephalus
megalocephalia
megalocephaly
congenital or acquired condition

large heart
cardiomegaly
megacardia
megalocardia

large intestine
enteromegalia
enteromegaly
megaloenteron
abnormal largeness of the intestine

large jaw
megagnathia
macrognathia

large limbs
macromelia
macromelus

large limbs (cont.)
megalomelia
abnormal size of one or more of the extremities

large liver
hepatomegaly
megalohepatia

large mouth
macrostomia

large nails
macronychia
megalonychosis
abnormally large fingernails or toenails

large nucleus
macronucleus
meganucleus

large penis
macropenis
macrophallus
megalopenis

large pill
bolus
also large volume of intra-venous fluid given rapidly

large rectum
megarectum

large sigmoid
macrosigmoid
megasigmoid

large spleen
splenomegaly
splenohepatomegalia
splenohepatomegaly
enlargement of spleen and liver

large stomach
macrogastric
megalogastria
megastria

large teeth
macrodont
macrodontia
megadont

large teeth (cont.)
megalodont
megalodontia

large toes
macrodactylia
macrodactylism
macrodactyly
megalodactylia
megalodactylism
megalodactly
    also applies to large fingers

large tongue
macroglossia
megaloglossia
pachyglossia

large writing
macrography
megalographia
    writing with very large letters

larva-killer
larvicide

larva second stage
cercaria

larynx artificial
laryngophantom

larynx disease
laryngopathy
    any disease of the larynx

larynx dryness
laryngoxerosis

larynx examination
laryngoscopy

larynx falling
laryngoptosis

larynx inflammation
laryngitis
laryngopharyngitis
    larynx and pharynx
laryngophthisis
    tuberculosis of the larynx
laryngotracheitis
    larynx and trachea

larynx inflammation (cont.)
laryngotracheobronchitis
    larynx, trachea and bronchi
perilaryngitis
    tissues surrounding the larynx
pharyngolaryngitis
    larynx and pharynx
rhinolaryngitis
    larynx and nose mucosa

larynx knife
laryngotome

larynx narrowing
laryngostenosis

larynx obstruction
laryngemphraxis

larynx operation
laryngectomy
laryngofissure
laryngotomy
cricothyroidotomy
intercricothyrotomy
hemilaryngectomy
laryngopharyngectomy
laryngoplasty
laryngostomy
laryngotracheotomy

larynx paralysis
laryngoparalysis
laryngoplegia
    paralysis of the laryngeal muscles

larynx recorder
laryngograph
laryngostroboscope

larynx softening
chondromalacia
laryngomalacia

larynx sounds
laryngophony
    voice sounds heard in auscultation of
    the larynx

larynx spasm
laryngismus

larynx spasmodic closure
glottidospasm
laryngospasm

larynx specialist
laryngologist
laryngoscopist

larynx study
laryngology
laryngorhinology
larynx and nose

larynx viewer
laryngoscope

laughter
risus

laughter inappropriate
cachinnation
immoderate and loud

lead monoxide
litharge

lead poisoning
plumbism
saturnism

leech
Hirudo medicinalis
leeches used in medicine for bleeding patients

left-eyed
sinistrocular

left-footed
sinistropedal

left-handed
sinistromanual

left-turning toward
levoversion

leg calf
sura
sural
muscular swelling of the back of the leg below the knee

leg cramp
systremma

leg excess
polyscelia
polyscelus
fetus born with more than two legs

leg lacking
monoscelous

leg largeness
macroscelia

leg shortness
brachyskelic

leg strength measurer
pedodynamometer
instrument to measure the muscular strength of the legs

lens bulging
lentiglobus

lens capsule
capsula lentis
phacocyst

lens capsule operation
phacocystectomy

lens displacement
phacocele
hernia of the crystalline lens of the eye

lens measurer
auxometer
axometer
axonometer
lensometer
phacometer*
*obsolete term

lens-shaped
lenticular
lentiform
phacoid

lens small
microlentia
microphakia
spherophakia

lens viewer
phacoscope
dark chamber for observing changes

96

leprosy hospital
leprosarium
lazaret
lazaretto

leprosy study
leprology

lesbianism
amor lesbicus
sapphism

leucine in urine
leucinuria

leukocyte counter
leukocytometer
glass slide ruled for counting white cells in a measured volume of blood

leukocyte deficiency
leukocytopenia
leukopenia

leukoma of cornea
exotropia
walleye

levulose in blood
levulosemia
presence of fructose in the circulating blood

levulose in urine
levulosuria

lewisite
chlorovinyldichloroarsine
poisonous warfare gas

lice
Pediculus

lice infestation
pediculation
pediculosis
presence of the parasites that live in the hair and feed on the blood

lice-killer
pediculicide

licorice
glycyrrhiza

lie detector
polygraph
psychogalvanometer

life development study
biogenesis
biogeochemistry

lifelessness
abiosis
abiotrophy
absence of life

ligament inflammation
desmitis
syndesmitis

ligament operation
syndesmopexy
syndesmoplasty
syndesmotomy

ligament study
syndesmology

ligament suture
syndesmorrhaphy

ligament-like
desmoid

light decomposing
photolysis
through the action of light
photolyte
product of light decomposition

light measurement
photometry

limb in excess
polymelia
polymelus
presence of supernumerary limbs or parts

limb lacking
ectromelia
ectromelus
lipomeria
monopodia
monopus

limb largeness
macromelia
macromelus
megalomelia

limbs malformed
melomelus
born with a rudimentary limb attached to a limb
peromelus
peromelia
peromely
born with malformed or deficient limbs

limb-pertaining
acral

limb sensation lacking
acroagnosis

limb smallness
micromelia
micromelus
nanomelia

limbs unequal
anisomelia
inequality between the two paired limbs

limbless
acolous

liniment
embrocation
rarely used term also meaning the application of

lionlike face
leontiasis

lip biting
cheilophagia
chilophagia

lips/cheeks
buccolabial

lips/chin
labiomental

lip eversion
eclabium

lip fusion/adhesion
syncheilia
synchilia
atresia of the mouth

lip inflammation
cheilitis
chilitis

lips lacking
acheilia
achilia

lip largeness
macrocheilia
macrochilia
abnormally enlarged lips

lip operation
cheilectomy
cheilotomy
cheiloplasty
chiloplasty
cheilostomatoplasty
chilostomatoplasty
labioplasty
rhinocheiloplasty
rhinochiloplasty

lip pain
cheilalgia
chilalgia

lip shortness
brachycheilia
brachychilia

lip silent movement
mussitation
observed in delirium and in semicoma

lip suture
cheilorrhaphy
chilorrhaphy

lip thickness/swelling
pachycheilia
pachychilia

liquid density measurer
densimeter

liquid expeller
hydragogue

liquid tension measurer
stalagmometer
instrument that measures the surface tension of liquids

liquid/gas in tissues
hydropneumatosis
accumulation of liquid and gas

lisping
sigmatism

lithic acid in urine
hyperlithuria
lithuria
excretion of large amounts of uric acid/ urates in the urine

liver atrophy
hepatatrophia
hepatatrophy

liver congestion
hepatohemia

liver destruction
hepatonecrosis
death of liver cells
hepatotoic
hepatotoxin
damaging to the liver

liver disease
hepatopathy

liver displacement
hepatoptosis

liver enlargement
hepatomegalia
hepatomegaly
megalohepatia
hepatosplenomegaly
splenohepatomegaly
liver and spleen
hepatonephromegaly
liver and kidneys

liver examination
hepatoscopy

liver hemorrhage
hepatorrhagia

liver hernia
hepatocele

liver inflammation
hepatitis
icterohepatitis
with jaundice
hepatosplenitis
liver and spleen
perihepatitis
peritoneum surrounding the liver
pleurohepatitis
liver and pleura

liver operation
hepatectomy
hepatotomy
hepatocholangioenterostomy
hepatocholangiostomy
hepatocholangiojejunostomy
hepatoduodenostomy
hepatolithectomy
hepatopexy
hepatostomy
hepaticostomy
hepaticoduodenostomy
hepaticoenterostomy
hepaticogastrostomy
hepaticolithotripsy

liver origin
hepatogenic
hepatogenous
formed in the liver

liver pain
hepatalgia
hepatodynia

liver pigmentation
hepatomelanosis
deep pigmentation of the liver

liver proximity
parahepatic

liver rupture
hepatorrhexis

liver softening
hepatomalacia

liver specialist
hepatologist

liver stone
hepatolith
hepatolithiasis

liver study
hepatology

liver suture
hepatorrhaphy

liver tumor
hepatoblastoma
hepatocarcinoma
hepatoma

liver x-ray
hepatography

liverlike
hepatoid

living in air
aerobic
aerophilic
aerophilous
organism that lives in the presence of oxygen

living without oxygen
anaerobic
organism that thrives best in the absence of oxygen

local anemia
hypoemia
ischemia

location abnormal
ectopic

lochial flow
lochiorrhea
lochiorrhagia

lockjaw
tetanus
trismus
painful tonic muscular contractions

long colon
dolichocolon

long-faced
dolichofacial
dolichoprosopic

long-headed
dolichocephalic
dolichocephalism
dolichocephaly
having a disproportionately long head

long-lived
macrobiote
macrobiotic

long-necked
dolichoderus

longevity
macrobiosis

longevity study
macrobiotics
study of the prolongation of life

loop
ansa

loss of appetite
anorexia

loss of body heat
thermolysis

loss of eyelashes
madarosis
milphosis

loss of memory
amnesia

loss of reading ability
alexia
inability to understand written symbols

loss of strength
adynamia
asthenia
debility

loss of taste
ageusia
ageustia

loss of touch/sensation
anesthesia
astereognosis
inability to recognize the form of an object by the touch
acroanesthesia
loss of feeling in the extremities

loss of vocal control
alalia
inability to control speech muscle

loss of voice
anaudia
aphonia

loving animals
zoophilia
zoophilism

loving children
pedophilia
excessive love for small children

loving elderly persons
gerontophilia

loving air
aerophil

low temperature measurer
cryometer

lower abdomen
hypogastrium

lower extremities only
acephalogaster
cojoined twin born with only the pelvis and legs

lower jaw
mandible
mandibula
submaxilla

lower jaw lacking
agnathia
agnathus
hemignathia
hypoagnathus
otocephalus

lower jaw small
hypognatous

lues
syphilis

lumbar puncture
rachicentesis

lumbar vertebra/sacrum angle
sacrovertebral angle

luminous perception
photopsia
photopsy
visual disorder where luminous rays are perceived

lump in throat
globus hystericus
spheresthesia

lumpy jaw
actinomycosis
actinophytosis

lung abscess
vomica
obsolete term

lung collapse
atelectasis

lung covering
pleura
the fine membrane covering each lung

lung disease
bronchopulmonary dysplasia
C>disorder seen in newborns
silicosis
progressive fibrosis due to inhilation of silica dust

lung flatulence
emphysema
accumulation of gas or air in any of the natural cavities

lung fungus disease
pneumonomycosis
pneumomycosis*
*obsolete term

lung gauge
  spirometer
    instrument used to measure lung capacity
  pneumatometer*
    *obsolete term

lung inflammation
  pneumonia
  pneumonitis
  bagassosis
  bird fancier's lung
  extrinsic allergic alveolitis
  farmer's lung
  pigeon breeder's lung
    hypersensitivity pneumonitis caused by repeated exposure to an allergen
  baritosis
    due to barium inhalation
  kaolinosis
    caused by inhaling clay dust
  pneumoconiosis
  pneumonoconiosis
    caused by dust
  pneumonomycosis
    caused by fungi

lung irritation
  byssinosis
  mill fever

lung lacking
  apneumia

lung operation
  lobectomy
  pneumectomy
  pneumonectomy
  pneumonotomy
  pneumotomy
  pulmonectomy
  pneumonopexy
  pneumopexy

lung puncture
  pneumocentesis
  pneumonocentesis
    paracentesis of the lung

lung suture
  pneumonorrhaphy

Lyme disease rash
  erythema chronicum migrans

lymph in blood
  lymphemia

lymph in urine
  chyluria
  lymphuria
    lymph or chyle

lymph cell/node
  lymphoblast
  lymphocele
  lymphocyte
  lymphocyst
  lymphonodus

lymph flow/escape
  lymphorrhea
    from ruptured, torn or cut lymphatic vessels

lymph formation
  lymphization
  lymphoblast
  lymphocerastism
  lymphocytopoiesis
  lymphogenesis
  lymphopoiesis

lymph inflammation
  adenitis
    of a gland or lymph node
  lymphadenitis
  lymphangitis
  lymphatitis
    of a lymph node
  lymphangiophlebitis
    lymph vessels and veins
  periangitis
    outside tissues around an artery, vein or lymph vessel
  perilymphangitis
    tissues around a lymph vessel

lymph lacking
  alymphia

lymph node
  lymphonodus

lymph node disease
adenopathy
lymphadenopathy
lymphopathy
any disease process affecting the lymph nodes or vessels

lymph node enlargement
hyperadenosis
lymphadema
lymphadenosis
lymphadenectasia*
lymphadenia*
*obsolete terms

lymph node/vessel x-ray
lymphadenography
lymphangiography
lymphography

lymph operation
lymphadenectomy
lymphangiectomy
lymphangioplasty
lymphangiotomy
lymphaticostomy
lymphoidectomy
lymphoplasty

lymph tumor
lymphadenoma
lymphoadenoma
lymphocytoma
lymphogranuloma
lymphomyeloma
lymphangiosarcoma
lymphoblastoma
lymphoepithelioma
lymphoma
lymphosarcoma
malignant forms of lymph tumors
lymphangioendothelioma
lymphangioma
lymphomyxoma
nonmalignant forms of lymph tumors

lymph vessel dilatation
lymphangiectasia
lymphangiectasis
lymphangiectatic

lymphatic system study
lymphangiology
lymphatology
lymphology
branch of medical science that pertains to the lymphatic system

magnesium/aluminum
magnalium
alloy containing the two metals

magnetism
mesmerism

maidenhead
hymen

malaria study
malariology

male birth
androgenous
giving birth to males

male reproduction
arrhenotocia

male sex disliked
apandria

male sterilization
deferentectomy
gonangiectomy
vasectomy

malnutrition
athrepsia
athrepsy
weakness due to lack of nourishment

malocclusion specialist
orthodontist

malocclusion study
orthodontics

mammary gland overgrowth
hypermastia
polymastia
   excessively large mammary glands

mammary gland smallness
hypomastia
hypomazia

mania for one thing
monomania

mania for writing
graphomania

mankind aversion
misanthropy
   aversion to people; hatred of mankind

manlike
android
anthropomorphic

many ancestors
polyphletic

marihuana
cannabis

marriage aversion
misogamy

marrow
medulla
   any soft, marrow-like structure

marrow cells stoppage
anakmesis

marrow fibrosis
myelofibrosis
myelosclerosis

marrow inflammation
myelitis

marshmallow root
althea

marshy
paludal

mask of pregnancy
chloasma

massage
massotherapy
sciage

massagist
masseur
male

masseuse
female

mastication insufficient
psomophagia
psomophagy
   swallow food without sufficient chewing

mastication measurer
phagodynamometer
   instrument to measure the force exerted in chewing

mastoid inflammation
mastoiditis

mastoid operation
mastoidectomy
mastoidotomy

maxillary sinus cavity
antronasal

measles
morbelli

measurement of body
anthropometry
   art of measuring the human body

meat poisoning
allantiasis
botulism

meatus operation
meatotomy
parotomy

median cerebellar lobe
ala lobuli centralis
   the lateral winglike projection of the central lobule of the cerebellum

mediastinum inflammation
mediastinitis
mediastinopericarditis

mediastinum operation
mediastinotomy

melancholia
barythymia

melanin in blood
melanemia

membrane
meninx
most often seen in pleural form as "meninges" of brain

membrane inflammation
serositis
of a serous membrane
serosynovitis
membrane and synovial fluid
synovitis
of a synovial membrane

membrane in urine
meninguria

memory acuteness
hypermnesia
extraordinary ability to recall

memory developing
mnemonics

memory divulgement
anamnesis
anamnestic
information obtained about one's past

memory impairment
dysmnesia
hypomnesia

memory loss
amnesia
amnesic
amnestic
ecmnesia
ability to recall only recent events

meninges hemorrhage
meningorrhagia

meninges inflammation
leptomeningitis
meningitis

meninges suture
meningeorrhaphy

meningococci in blood
meningococcemia

menses
catamenia
emmenia

menses first appearance
menophania

menses retention
menoschesis
suppression of menstruation

menstrual disorder
paramenia
xeromenia

menstrual flow deficiency
hypomenorrhea
oligomenorrhea

menstrual flow excessive
hypermenorrhea
menorrhagia

menstrual pain
dysmenorrhea
menorrhalgia
difficult and painful menstruation

menstrual stoppage
amenorrhea
menopause
menostasia
menostasis

menstruation beginning
menarche
for the first time

menstruation inducer
emmenagogue

menstruation irregular
menoxenia
paramenia

menstruation lacking
amenia
amenorrhea

menstruation life
menacme
interval during a woman's lifetime for menses

menstruation prolonged
hypermenorrhea
menostaxis

menstruation substitute
menocelis
type of vicarious menstruation with spots on the skin when menstruation fails

mental alertness
prothymia

mental confusion
obfuscation
psychataxia

mental deficiency
amentia
ament*
*obsolete term for a mentally retarded person

mental disorder
neophrenia
psychoneurosis
psychoplegia
psychorrhexis
psychosis

mental development
psychogenesis
psychogeny

mental disease
psychopathia
psychopathy
an old, inexact term referring to a pattern of inappropriate behavior

mental disease category
psychonosology
classification of diseases

mental strain
psychentonia

mental testing
psychometrics
psychometry

mercury
hydrargyrum

mercury poisoning
hydrargyria
hydrargyrism

mesentery fixation
mesenteriopexy
mesopexy

mesentery suture
mesenteriorrhaphy
mesorrhaphy
suture of the layer of peritoneum attached to the abdominal wall

metabolism measurer
metabolimeter

metacarpal operation
metacarpectomy
excision of one or all of the metacarpal bones of the hand

metaphysis inflammation
metaphysitis

metatarsal operation
metatarsectomy

metatarsal pain
metatarsalgia

metatarsal/metacarpal shortness
brachymetapody

methemoglobin in blood
methemoglobinemia

methemoglobin in urine
methemoglobinuria

microbe-killer
microbicide
a germicide or antiseptic

microbe study
microbiology

middle ear
auris media

midwifery
obstetrics
tocology

migraine
hemicephalalgia
hemicrania

mild
benign
mitis

mild smallpox
alastrim
caused by a less virulent strain of virus

milk albumin
lactalbumin

milk arrester
antigalactic

milk coagulatory
chymosin
eenase
rennet
rennin
present in the chief cells of the gastric tubules

milk cure
galactotherapy
lactotherapy

milk deficiency
oligogalactia

milk duct dilatation
ampulla lactifera
sinus lactiferi

milk in excess
polygalactia

milk fat measurer
galactometer
lactocrit
lactometer
instrument to determine the specific gravity of milk as an indication of its fat content

milk flow
galactorrhea
lactorrhea

milk flow stoppage
agalorrhea

milk lacking
agalactia
agalactosis
agalactous

milk leg
phlegmasia alba dolens
extreme swelling due to thrombosis of the veins

milk protein
lactoprotein

milk secretion lower
hypogalactia

milk with sugar excess
saccharogalactorrhea

milky diarrhea
chylorrhea
the flow or discharge of chyle

milky urine
chyluria
galacturia

mind
psychic
psychical

mind alertness
eunoia
denoting a normal mental state

mind altering
psychoactive
psychopharmaceutical
psychostimulant
psychotogen
psychogenic
psychotomimetic
psychotropic

mind development/origin
psychogenic
psychogenesis

mind development/origin (cont.)
psychogenetic
of mental origin or causation

mind specialist
psychoanalyst
psychiatrist
psychotherapist

mind stimulant
psychogogic
acting as a stimulant to the emotions

mind study
psychiatry
psychoanalysis
psychodynamics
psychology
psychonomy
psychopathology
psychotherapy

mind treatment
psychotherapy

minor lip inflammation
nymphitis

minute measurer
acribometer
instrument to measure very small objects

miscarriage
abortion

mixable
miscible

molar-shaped
molariform

molecule largeness
macromolecule

monocyte largeness
macromonocyte
an unusually large cell

mood disorder
dysthymia

mood swings
cyclothymia

mortification of tissue
gangrene
necrosis
sphacelation
sphacelism
sphacelous

mother-killer
matricide

motion in excess
acrocinesia
acrocinesis
excessive movement

motion sickness
kinesia

motion study
kinetics

mouth disease
stomatopathy
stomatosis
stomatomycosis
fungal disease

mouth disinfection
stomatocatharsis

mouth dryness
xerostomia

mouth hemorrhage
stomatomenia
stomatorrhagia
stomenorrhagia
bleeding from the gums

mouth inflammation
stomatitis

mouth lacking
astomia
astomatous
astomous
opocephalus
congenital absence

mouth operation
stomatoplasty
stomatotomy

mouth pain
stomatalgia
stomatodynia

mouth proximity
adoral

mouth smallness
microstomia

mouth/teeth study
stomatology
study of the structures, functions and diseases of the mouth

mouth ulcer
noma
stomatonecrosis
stomatonoma

mouth viewer
stomatoscope

movement difficulty/disorder
dyscinesia
dyskinesia

movement repetition
palicinesia
palikinesia

movement slow
bradykinesia

mucous deficiency
amyxia
amyxorrhea

mucous discharge
blenorrhea
myxorrhea

mucuslike
myxoid

mud treatment
pelopathy
pelotherapy
application of mud, peat, moor or clay to parts of the body

mumps
parotiditis
parotitis

murderous tendency
hemothymia

muscle cell
myoblast
myocyte

muscle contraction
clonus
alternating with relaxation
myoclonus
shocklike contractions
myodynamia
myodynamics
denotes muscular strength

muscle degeneration
muscular dystrophy

muscle deterioration
amyotrophia
amyotrophy
myoatrophy
myocerosis
myodermia
myolysis
myonecrosis

muscle disease
myonosus
myopathy
any abnormal condition or disease of muscular tissue

muscle dislocation
myectopia
myectopy

muscle edema
myoedema

muscle fiber sheath
myolemma
sarcolemma

muscle fiber tumor
rhabdomyoma
*myoma striocellulare**
*obsolete term

muscle flaccidity
hypotonia

muscle formation
myogenesis

muscle formation lacking
amyoplasia

muscle inflammation
myositis
myocelitis
abdominal muscles
myocellulitis
muscles and cellular tissues
myofibrositis
perimysium
perimyositis
tissues around the muscles
polymyositis
several muscles
pyomyositis
accompanied by pus

muscle measurer
myochronoscope
timing muscle impulse
myodynamometer
determine strength
myograph
timing contractions
myokinesimeter
myometer
myophone
reflexometer
force required to produce movement

muscle operation
myectomy
myoplasty
myotomy
myotenotomy
scalenectomy
scalenotomy
tenomyotomy
tenontomyotomy

muscle origin
myogenetic
myogenic
originating in or starting from muscle

muscle pain
myalgia

muscle pain (cont.)
myocelialgia
myodynia
myoneuralgia
myosalgia
polymyalgia

muscle paralysis
myoparalysis
myoparesis

muscle quivering
kymatism
myoclonus
myokymia
irregular spasm or twitching of the muscles

muscle rigidity
anochlesia
catalepsy

muscle separation
myodiastasis

muscle softness
myomalacia
pathological softening of muscle tissue

muscle specialist
myologist

muscle study
myology

muscle tumor
leiomyoma
myoblastoma
myocytoma
myoepithelioma
myofibroma
myolemma
myolipoma
myoma
myoneuroma
rhabdomyoma

muscle twitching
myoclonus
chronic spasm of one or a group of muscles
myokyma

muscle twitching (cont.)
myopalmus
irregular twitching of most of the muscles

muscle weakness
myasthenia

muscular atrophy
amyotrophia
amyotrophic
amyotrophy

muscular dystrophy
dystrophia myotonica
myodystrophia
myodystrophy

muscular hypertrophy
myopachynis

muscular impulse failure
adromia
lack of impulse transmission in nerves or muscles

muscular incoordination
amyotaxia
amyotaxy
ataxia

muscular sense lost
muscular anesthesia

muscular strength measurer
dynamometer

muscular tone lacking
amyotonia
myatonia
myatony
abnormal extensibility of a muscle

mushroom poisoning
muscarinism
mycetism
mycetismus

mushroom-shaped
fungiform
fungoid

mushroom study
*mycology*i

mushy
pultaceous

musical fascination
melomania

musical recognition loss
amusia
loss of ability to understand music

mustard gas
dichlorodiethylsulfide

mutualism
symbiosis
living together in harmony

myelin destruction
myelinoclasis

myelocytes in blood
myelemia
myelocytosis

myocardium inflammation
myocarditis

myoglobin in blood
myoglobinemia

myoglobin in urine
myoglobinuria

N

nail
unguis

nail atrophy
onychatrophia
onychatrophy

nail biting
onychophage
onychophagia
onychophagy
one who bites

nail blackness
melanonychia
   condition where nails of the fingers or
   toes turn black

nail breaking
onychoclasis

nail component
keratin

nail curvature
gryposis unguium
onychogryposis
   abnormal curvature

nail disease
onychopathy
onychosis

nail displacement
onychoptosis
   downward displacement

nail dystrophy
dystrophia unguium

nails in excess
polyunguia
   having more than the normal number of
   nails

nail fungal disease
onychomycosis
tinea ungium

nail hardening
scleronychia
   also with thickness

nail hypertrophy
onychauxis

nail inflammation
onychia
onychitis
onyxitis
   inflammation of the matrix
onchyia lateralis
paronychia
   marginal inflammation accompanied by
   pus

nail inflammation (cont.)
perionychia
perionyxis
   inflammation surrounding the nail

nail ingrowing
onychocryptosis

nails lacking
anonychia
anonychosis

nails largeness
macronychia
megalonychosis

nail in layers
onychoschizia

nail matrix
onychostroma

nail-moon
lunula
   the white moon-shaped part at the base
   of a nail

nail operation
onychectomy
onychotomy

nail smallness
micronychia

nail softness
onychomalacia
   abnormal softness

nail splitting
onychorrhexis
schizonychia

nail thickened
pachyonychia

nail thickened/curved
onychogryphosis
onychogryposis

nail whiteness
leukonychia
leukopathia unguis
   caused by air beneath the nail

nape of neck
nucha

narcotic craving
narcomania

narrowing
stenosis

narrowing of an opening
arctation
stenosis

narrowness of head
stenocephalia
stenocephalic
stenocephaly

nasal
rhinal

nasal passage dryness
xeromycteria
pertaining to the nose

nasal plug
rhinobyon

nasal proximity
paranasal
located near the nose

nasal voice
rhinolalia
rhinophonia

nasopharynx
epipharynx
pars nasalis pharyngis

nature cure
naturopathy
using physical methods

nausea
sicchasia

navel
omphalos
umbilicus

navel inflammation
omphalitis
inflammation of the umbilicus and surrounding parts

navel operation
omphalectomy
omphalotomy
omphalotripsy

navel region
parumbilical

navel varicosity
varicomphalus

near the mouth
adoral

near a nerve
adnerval
adneural

near the sternum
adsternal

nearsightedness
myope
individual concerned
myopia
the condition

neck-back
nape
nucha
back of the neck

neck cleft
tracheloschisis
congenital fissure

neck/face
cervicofacial

neck/head lacking
atrachelocephalus
fetus with head and neck either missing or not developed

neck pain
trachelodynia

neck spasm
trachelism
trachelismus
spasmodic contraction of the neck muscles

neck stiffness
loxia
torticollis
wryneck

needle-shaped
acicular

nerve activity
neurergic

nerve acupuncture
neuronyxis

nerve antagonist
sympatholytic
adrenergic nerve blocking agent

nerve-bundle sheath
epineurium
envelops a fasciculus of nerves
perineurium
envelops each funiculus of a nerve fiber

nerve cell
axon
neuroblast
neuroblastoma
neurocyte
neuron
*neuraxon**
*obsolete term

nerve crushing
neurotripsy

nerve destruction
neurocytolysis
neurolysis

nerve disease
neuropathy
any disease of the nervous system

nerve disease sufferer
neuropath

nerve disease treatment
neuriatria
neuriatry

nerve displacement
neurectopia
neurectopy

nerve energy
neurodynamic

nerve energy lacking
aneuria

nerve exhaustion
neurasthenia
particularly when due to mental strain

nerve fiber divider
leukotome

nerve fibrous sheath
neurilemma
neurolemma

nerve formation
neurogenesis

nerve impulse failure
adromia
absence of impulse transmission in nerves or muscles

nerve inflammation
mononeuritis
affecting only one nerve
neuritis
involving the nerves in general
neurochorioretinitis
chorioretinitis and optic neuritis combined
neurochoroiditis
choroid body and the optic nerve
neurodermatitis
neurodermatosis
skin inflammation where nerves are involved
neuromyelitis
involves spinal cord
neuromyositis
involves nerves and muscles
neuromyelitis optica
optic nerve and white/gray matter of the brain
neuroretinitis
optic nerve and retina
multiple neuritis
polyneuritis
inflammation of several nerves

nerve inflammation (cont.)
  radiculitis
    nerve roots involved
  actinoneuritis
  radioneuritis
    inflammation caused by exposure to x-rays

nerve operation
  neurectomy
  neuroectomy
  neuroplasty
  neurotomy
  neurotripsy
  neurexeresis
  neuroanastomosis
  radicotomy
  rhizotomy
  splanchnicectomy
  splanchnicotomy

nerve pain
  neuralgia
  neurodynia
    pain in general
  polyneuralgia
    involving several nerves

nerve proximity
  adnerval
  adneural

nerve specialist
  neurologist
  neurosurgeon

nerve stimulant
  analeptic
    central nervous system stimulant

nerve stretching
  neurectasia
  neurectasis
  neurectasy

nerve study
  neurology

nerve suture
  neurorrhaphy
  neurosuture
    joining two parts of a divided nerve

nerve tissue softness
  neuromalacia

nerve tumor
  neurilemoma
  neurinoma
  neuroschwannoma
  schwannoma
  neurocytoma
  ganglioneuroma
  neurofibroma
  neurosarcoma

nerve treatment
  neurotherapeutics
  neurotherapy
    treatment of nervous disorders

nerve/vein network
  plexus

network
  plexus
  reticulum

nettle
  urtica

nettle rash
  urticaria

neurosis localized
  toponeurosis

never borne children
  nullipara

newborn measurer
  mecometer
    instrument for measuring newborn infants

newness aversion
  misoneism
    dislike of changes

night blindness
  nyctalopia

night lover
  nyctophilia
  scotophilia
    condition of giving preference to darkness

night pain
nyctalgia
    occurs only at night

nightmare
incubus

nipple erection
thelerthism

nipples in excess
hyperthelia
polythelism
    congenital presence of more than usual
    number

nipple hemorrhage
thelorrhagia

nipple inflammation
mammillitis
thelitis

nipples lacking
athelia

nipple operation
mammilliplasty
theleplasty
    plastic surgery of the nipple and areola

nipple pain
thelalgia

nipple smallness
microthelia

nipplelike
papillary

nitrates in urine
nitrituria

nitrogen in blood
hyperazotemia
    excessive amount

nitrogen measurer
nitrometer
    instrument to determine amount of nitro-
    gen given off in a chemical reaction

nitrogen in urine
hyperazoturia
    excessive amount

nodes on bone
Heberden's nodes
tuberculum arthriticum
    growths on the end of the phalanges
    (fingers) seen in osteoarthritis

nodes on hair
monilethrix
    disease causing the appearance of
    nodes

noise pain
odynacusis
    discomfort caused by noises

noise-unit
decibel

normal blood pressure
normotensive
normotonic

normal blood volume
normovolemia

normal color
normochromatic

normal calcium in blood
normocalcemia

normal erythrocyte
normocyte
    normal cell size

normal erythrocyte color
normochromia

normal glucose in blood
normoglycemia

normal position
normotopia

normal potassium in blood
normokalemia
    normal level of potassium in the blood

normal pregnancy
uterogestation

normal temperature
normothermia

normoblast largeness
macroblast
macronormoblast
promegaloblast
pronormoblast

nose acne
rhinophyma
a type appearing on the nose

nose bleeding
epistaxis
rhinorrhagia

nose prominent
rhinokyphosis
refers to the bridge

nose constriction
rhinocleisis
rhinostenosis

nose discharging
rhinorrhea

nose disease
rhinopathy
general term for any disorder of the nose

nose hair
vibrissa

nose hemorrhage
epistaxis
rhinorrhagia

nose inflammation
coryza
inflammation of the mucous membrane
nasopharyngitis
inflammation of the nasal passages and pharynx
pansinuitis
pansinusitis
inflammation of all paranasal tissues
pharyngorhinitis
inflammation of the pharynx and nasal membranes
rhinomycosis
fungal infection

nose inflammation (cont.)
rhinitis
inflammation of the nasal membranes
rhinoantritis
inflammation of the nasal membranes and maxillary sinus
rhinolaryngitis
inflammation of the mucosa and larynx
rhinopharyngitis
inflammation of nose and pharynx
sinusitis
inflammation of the nasal cavities

nose inflator
rhineurynter
elastic bag inflated after insertion into the nose

nose knife
spokeshave
surgical instrument

nose lacking
arhinia
arrhinia

nose/lips
nasolabial

nose long and thin
leptorrhine

nose measurer
rhinomanometer
rhinomanometry
instrument to measure degree of nasal obstruction

nose obstruction
rhinocleisis

nose operation
rhinoplasty
rhinotomy
rhinocheiloplasty
septectomy
septotomy
sinusotomy
turbinectomy
turbinotomy

nose pain
rhinalgia
rhinodynia

nose pointed
oxyrhine
having a sharp pointed nose

nose purulent discharge
ozena
rhinitis purulenta

nose running
rhinorrhea
discharge from the nasal mucous membrane

nose shortness
brachyrhinia
shortness of nose in general
brachyrhynchus
shortness of nose and maxilla

nose specialist
rhinologist

nose stone
rhinodacryolith
rhinolith
rhinolite
rhinolithiasis
rhinopharyngolith

nose study
rhinology
laryngorhinology

nose viewer
nasopharyngoscope
instrument to examine nose and pharynx
rhinoscope
instrument to examine nasal passages

nose voice
rhinophonia
voice with nasal quality

nose wing
alinasal

nuclear membrane
karyotheca

numbness
obdormition
due to pressure on the sensory nerve

nutmeg
myristica

nutrition
tropism

nutrition disorder
trophonosis
trophopathy

nutritive
alible

nympha
labium minus

numph inflammation
nymphitis

nympha operation
nymphectomy
nymphotomy
surgical procedure on the minor lips of the vulva

nymph swelling
nymphoncus

O

obesity
adiposis
condition of fat accumulation

objects falsely magnified
macroesthesia
sensation that objects are larger than they are

oblique amputation
loxotomy
in an oblique section

obscenity
coprolalia
coprophrasia
involuntary utterance of obscenities

obscure origin
cryptogenic
refers to source of disease

obstetric tool
vectis

obstruction
emphraxis
of the sweat glands

ocular muscle paralysis
ophthalmoplegia

ohm measurer
ohmmeter

oil gravity measurer
eleometer
oleometer

oily
oleaginous

old age
senium
especially the debility of the aged

old age study
geriatrics

old skin
geroderma
gerodermia

olefiant gas
ethylene

olfactory organs lacking
cyclencephalia
cyclencephaly
cyclocephalia
cyclocephaly
congenital fusion of the two cerebral
hemispheres

omentum
epiploic
omental

omentum hernia
enterepiplocele
enteroepiplocele

omentum lacking
anepiploic

omentum operation
omentectomy
omentopexy
*epiploectomy**
*obsolete term

omentum suture
omentorrhaphy
*epiplorrhaphy**
*obsolete term

one child
primiparous
uniparous
female who has had only one child

one-fingered/toed
monodactylism
monodactyly
a single digit on hand or foot

one-footed
monopodia
monopus
sympus monopus
born with only one foot or leg

one-sided pain
hemialgia

one-track mind
monoideism
monomania
dwelling excessively on a single subject

ooze
transude
liquid through a membrane

open country lover
agromania
having an excessive desire to be isolat-
ed or in open country

operation of...
(see under specific site)

opium alkaloids
codeine
morphine
papaverine
thebaine
tritopine

opium tincture
laudanum

opposite therapy
heteropathy
method of treating diseases by creating opposite or different conditions

oppositely situated
antipodal

optical image distortion
anamorphosis
correction by glasses

orbit operation
orbitotomy
of the eye orbit

organ/gland cells
parenchyma
distinguishing cells of a gland or organ

organ correlation
synergy
among different organs of the body

organ displacement
anteversion
dystopia
forward displacement of any organ

organ formation
organogenesis

organ lacking
ectrogeny
loss or congenital absence of all or part of an organ

organ malposition
ectopia
ectopic
ectopy
heterotopia
heterotopic

organ measurer
oncometer
instrument used to measure the size and configuration of organs

organic development
organogenesis
organogeny

organic tissue dissolution
histolysis

orifice muscle
sphincter
surrounding an opening

orifice muscle operation
sphincterectomy
sphincteroplasty
sphincterotomy

origin-equaled
isogenous
having the same origin

orthopedic appliances
orthopraxis
orthopraxy
employment of artificial appliances

osmotic pressure unequal
anisotonic

ossified cancer
osteocarcinoma

ossified fetus
ostembryon
obsolete term for lithopedion

outbreeding
exogamy
cross-fertilization

outgrowth
excrescence

outward appearance
physiognomy
physical characteristics and general appearance

ovarian abscess
pyo-ovarium

ovarian pregnancy
ovariocyesis

ovary development lacking
ovarian agenesis

ovary hardening
sclero-oophoritis

ovary hernia
ovariocele

ovary inflammation
oophoritis
ovaritis
   inflammation of the ovary in general
paraoophoritis
perisalpingo-ovaritis
perioophorosalpingitis
   inflammation of the tissues around the
   ovary and oviduct
perioophoritis
periovaritis
   inflammation of the ovary, peritoneum,
   and surrounding tissues

ovary operation
oophorectomy
ovariectomy
oophorosalpingectomy
ovariosalpingectomy
oophoroplasty
oophorohysterectomy
ovariohysterectomy
oophorostomy
ovariostomy
ovariotomy
panhysterosalpingo-oophorectomy
salpingo-oophorectomy
salpingo-oothecectomy
salpingoovariectomy

ovary pain
oarialgia
ovarialgia
ovarian neuralgia
ovariodysneuria

ovary puncture
ovariocentesis
   also applies to puncture of a cyst

ovary rupture
ovariorrhexis

ovary/testis combined
ovotestis
   a form of hermaphroditism

ovary or testis lacking
agonadism
   or absence of functions

ovary and tube inflamed
adnexitis
annexitis

ovary tumor
arrhenoblastoma
mesonephroma

ovary and uterine tube
adnexa uteri

ovary varicosity
ovarian varicocele

overdevelopment
hypertrophia
hypertrophy
   over development of an organ or body
   part not due to tumor

overfeeding
hyperalimentation
hypernutrition
supernutrition

overflowing tears
epiphora
   accumulation of tears in the eyes

overlapping
imbrication
   layers of tissue in surgical suturing

oviduct hernia
salpingocele
   protrusion in general
salpingo-oophorocele
   protrusion of an ovary and oviduct

oviduct inflammation
parasalpingitis
   inflammation of the tissues surrounding
   an oviduct

oviduct operation

panhysterosalpingectomy
hysterosalpingectomy
hysterosalpingooophorectomy
hysterosalpingostomy
oophorosalpingectomy
ovariosalpingectomy
panhysterosalpingooophorectomy

oviduct pus

pyosalpinx
accumulation of pus in an oviduct

ovum elastic envelope

oolemma
zona pellucida

oxalates in blood excessive

oxalemia

oxalic acid in urine

hyperoxaluria
oxaluria
also applies to presence of oxylates

oyster poisoning

ostreotoxism

P

pace measurer

pedometer
podometer
instrument that measures the distance walked

pain of abdominal gas

tympanism
tympanites

pain of Achilles tendon

achillodynia

pain allaying

analgia
analgic
analgesic
analgetic

pain of anus

proctalgia
proctodynia
sphincteralgia
pain at the anus or in the rectum

pain in arm

brachialgia

pain in back

dorsalgia

pain of bladder

cystalgia

pain of body

pantalgia
affecting all parts

pain of bones

ostealgia
osteodynia

pain of breast

mammalgia
mastalgia
mastodynia
mazodynia

pain of burning sensation

causalgia
persistent severe burning sensation of the skin

pain in buttocks

pygalgia

pain of cartilage

xiphodynia
xyphoidalgia

pain in cheek area

carotidynia
carotodynia
pain caused by pressure on the carotid artery

122

pain of chest
thoracodynia
thoracomyodynia

pain of clitoris
clitoralgia

pain of coccyx
coccyalgia
coccygodynia

pain of cold
cryalgesia
psychralgia
psychroalgia
produced by application of cold

pain, constricting
angina

pain of dental pulp
pulpalgia

pain of ears
otalgia
otodynia
otoneuralgia

pain referred
synalgia
pain away from the injured part

pain of epigastrium
epigastralgia

pain of esophagus
esophagalgia

pain excessive sensitivity
hyperalgesia
morbid sensitivity to pain

pain of the extremities
melagra
melalgia
acrostealgia
pain in bones of extremities

pain of eye
ophthalmalgia
ophthalmodynia
ophthalmagra

pain of face
prosoponeuralgia

pain of foot
podalgia
pododynia

pain as girdle sensation
zonesthesia
sensation similar to that produced by the tightness of a girdle

pain of gland
adenalgia
dacryoadenalgia

pain of groin
inguinodynia

pain of head
cephalgia
cephalalgia
cephalodynia
encephalalgia
headache
algopsychalia
phrenalgia
psychalgalia
psychalgia
usually caused by a depressed condition rather than physical causes

pain of heart
cardialgia
cardiodynia

pain of heat
thermalgesia
thermoalgesia
excessive sensibility to heat

pain of heel
calcaneodynia
talsalgia

pain of hip
coxalgia
coxodynia

pain in inguinal zone
bubonalgia

pain insensitivity
analgesia
analgia
  inability to feel pain in any parts

pain of intestine
enteralgia
enterodynia
gastroenteralgia

pain of joint
arthralgia
arthralgic
arthrodynia
arthrodynic
  severe pain in a joint, especially one not
  inflammatory in nature

pain of kidney
nephralgia

pain of knee
gonalgia
gonagra

pain lacking
anodynia
  absence of pain in a body part

pain of legs
skelalgia

pain of lips
cheilalgia
chilalgia

pain of liver
hepatalgia
hepatodynia

pain measurer
algesimeter
  instrument to measure acuteness of
  pain
dolorimeter
  measures sensitivity to pain
ponograph
  measures progressive fatigue of a contracting muscle

pain of menstruation
dysmenorrhea
menorrhalgia

pain of metatarsus
metatarsalgia

pain in missing limb
phantom limb
  feeling pain in an amputated limb

pain of mouth
stomatalgia
stomatodynia

pain of muscle
myalgia
  muscular pain

pain of neck
cervicodynia
trachelodynia
torticollis
wryneck

pain of nerves
neuralgia
neurodynia
polyneuralgia

pain at night
nyctalgia

pain of nipple
thelalgia

pain of noise
odynacusis
  hypersensitiveness of the ear

pain of nose
rhinalgia
rhinodynia

pain on one side of body
hemialgia

pain of ovary
oarialgia
ovarialgia
ovarian neuralgia
ovariodysneuria

pain of pharynx
pharyngalgia
pharyngodynia
  pain in the region of the throat

pain of pleura
pleuralgia
pleurodynia

pain of pylorus
pyloralgia

pain of rectum
proctalgia
proctodynia
rectalgia

pain reliever
analgesic
anodyne
antineuralgic
relieves pain of a nerve

pain of rheumatism
rheumatalgia

pain of ribs
costalgia
intercostal neuralgia
pleurodynia
subcostalgia

pain of sacrum
sacralgia
sacrodynia

pain of scapula
scapulalgia
pain in the region of the shoulder blades

pain sensitivity
algesia
algesic
algetic

pain sensitivity in excess
hyperalgesia
hyperalgia

pain severe
megalgia

pain of skin
dermatalgia
dermatodynia
erythromelalgia
rodonalgia

pain in sleep
hypnalgia
experienced during sleep

pain source
algogenesia
algogenesis

pain of spleen
splenalgia
splenodynia

pain of stomach
gastralgia
gastroenteralgia
cardialgia
peratodynia

pain from strong light
photalgia
photodynia
pain experienced when under the intensity of strong light

pain sudden
twinge
a sudden sharp pain of short duration

pain suffocating
angina
spasmodic, choking sensation

pain in tarsus of foot
tarsalgia

pain of teeth
dentalgia
odontalgia
odontodynia
toothache
aerodontalgia
toothache due to high altitude flying

pain of tendon
tenalgia
tenodynia
tenontodynia

pain of thigh
meralgia

pain of tibia
tibialgia

125

pain of tongue
glossalgia
glossodynia

pain on touching objects
haphalgesia
pain or unpleasant sensation caused by touch

pain of trachea
trachealgia
trachelodynia

pain of urethra
urethralgia

pain of urinary bladder
cystalgia

pain of urinary tract
urocrisia
urocrisis

pain of urination
dysuria
urodynia
difficulty or pain when urinating

pain of uterus
hysteralgia
hysterodynia
metralgia
metrodynia
uteralgia

pain of vagina
colpalgia
vaginodynia
vaginismus
vulvismus

pain of vertebrae
spondylalgia
spondylodynia

pain of viscera
visceralgia
pain in any of the internal organs

painless death
euthanasia

palate cleft
uranoschisis

palate high/narrow
hypsistaphilia

palate inflammation
palatitis

palate operation
palatoplasty
staphylectomy
staphylotomy
uranoplasty
uranostaphyloplasty
uvulectomy

palate paralysis
palatoplegia
of the soft palate

palate pendulum
uvula
fleshy conical mass located above the back of the tongue

palate suture
palatorrhaphy
staphylorrhaphy
uranorrhaphy
uranostaphyloplasty
uranostaphylorrhaphy

pale urine
achromaturia
lacking pigmentation

paleness of skin
achromia
achromasia
due to lack of pigment

palm of hand
thenar
vola
volar

palmar vesicles
cheiropompholyx
chiropompholyx
dyshidria
dishidrosis
pompholyx
blisters that appear on the palms of the hands and soles of the feet

126

palpable vibration
  fremitus

pancreas calculus
  pancreatolith
  pancreolith

pancreas disease
  pancreatopathy
  pancreopathy

pancreas inflammation
  pancreatitis
  peripancreatitis
    inflammation of the tissues surrounding the pancreas

pancreas lacking
  apancrea
  apancreatic

pancreas operation
  pancreatectomy
  pancreectomy
  pancreaticoduodenostomy
  pancreatoduodenostomy
  pancreatojejunostomy
  pancreaticolithotomy
  pancreatoduodenectomy
  pancreatolithectomy
  pancreatolithotomy
  pancreolithotomy
  pancreatomy
  pancreatotomy

pancreas proximity
  parapancreatic
    near the pancreas

pancreatic extract
  insulin
    Iletin®

pancreatic juice lacking
  achylia pancreatica

panic attack
  unreasoning anxiety
    accompanied by fear

panting
  hyperpnea
  polypnea

paralysis of bladder
  cystoparalysis
  cystoplegia

paralysis of extremities
  acroparalysis

paralysis of eye muscles
  ophthalmoplegia

paralysis of Intestines
  adynamic ileus
  enteroplegia
    usually as the result of peritonitis or shock

paralysis of legs
  paraparesis
  paraplegia
  paraplegic
  paraplegy

paralysis of limbs
  quadriplegia
  tetraplegia
    paralysis of all four extremities

paralysis of one side of body
  hemiparesis
  hemiplegia
  monoplegia

paralysis on two sides
  diplegia
  diplegic
    affecting equally corresponding parts on both sides of the body

paralysis partial
  monoparesis
    on one part of the body only

parasite absorber
  parasitotropic
    substance in the blood that absorbs parasites

parasite affinity
  parasitotropism
  parasitotropy

parasite in blood
  parasitemia

parasite disease
parasitosis
infestation with or any disease caused
by parasites

parasite fear
parasitophobia

parasite growth
parasitogenesis

parasite-killer
parasiticide

parasite specialist
parasitologist

parasite study
helminthology
parasitology

parenchyma inflammation
parenchymatitis
inflammation of the specific cells of a
gland or organ

parovarium inflammation
parovaritis

parrot fever
psittacosis

part defective or lacking
aplasia
congenital condition

parturition difficult
dystocia
parodynia

parturition normal
eutocia

parturition first time
primipara
primigravida
primiparity
first pregnancy

passage closing
stegnosis

patch/spot
tache

patella operation
patellectomy
removal

patella shaped
patelliform

pathology of extremities
acropathology

pea-shaped
pisiform

peace of mind
ataraxia
calmness or tranquility

Peale pill
phencyclidine (PCP)

peanut oil
arachis oil

peanut oil acid
arachic acid
arachidic acid

pear-shaped
piriform
pyriform

pearl-like
nacreous
resembling mother-of-pearl

peeling off
exfoliation
also denotes scaling off

pelvis measurer
pelvimeter
pelvimetry

pelvis narrowness
leptopellic

pelvis operation
pelvilithotomy
pelviolithotomy
pelviotomy

pelvis viewer
pelviscope
instrument for examining the interior of
the pelvis

penis
membrum virile
penile
phallic
phallus

penis deformity
hypospadias
urethra opens on the ventral side of the penis
paraspadias
urethra opens on one side of the penis
phallocampsis
curvature of the erect penis
phallocrypsis
dislocation and retraction

penis discharge
phallorrhea

penis hemorrhage
phallorrhagia

penis inflammation
balanitis
balanoposthitis

penis largeness
macropenis
megalopenis

penis operation
penotomy
phallectomy
phalloplasty
phallotomy

penis pain
phallalgia
phallodynia

penis pulling
peotillomania
manifestation of a nervous disorder

penis shaped
phalloid

penis smallness
micropenis
microphallus

penis tumor/swelling
phalloncus

penis worship
phallicism
phallism

pentose in urine
pentosuria

perception defective
imperception
inability to form a mental picture of an object

perception lacking
agnea
agnosia
inability to recognize by various sensory impressions
auditory agnosia
inability to recognize by sound
optic agnosia
inability to recognize by vision
tactile agnosia
inability to recognize by touch

pericardial sac fluid
pneumohydropericardium
air and fluid in the pericardial sac

pericardium inflammation
pericarditis
inflammation of the pericardium
pleuropericarditis
inflammation of pleura and pericardium
pyopericarditis
inflammation accompanied by pus

pericardium operation
pericardectomy
pericardiectomy
pericardiostomy
pericardiotomy

pericardium puncture
pericardiocentesis

pericardium pus
pyopneumopericardium
pus and gas or air in the pericardium

pericardium suture
pericardiorrhaphy

perineal hernia
perineocele

perineum operation
perineoplasty
perineotomy

perineum suture
perineorrhaphy

perineurium inflammation
perineuritis
inflammation of the connective tissue surrounding nerve fibers

periodontal inflammation
pericementitis
periodontitis

periosteum inflammation
parosteitis
parostitis

periosteum operation
periosteotomy

peritoneal cavity gas/air
aeroperitoneum
aeroperitonia
pyopneumoperitoneum

peritoneum disease
peritoneopathy
any disease or disorder of the peritoneum

peritoneum inflammation
pachyperitonitis
thickening of the peritoneum due to inflammation
pericolitis
pericolonitis
inflammation of tissues surrounding the colon
peritonitis
general inflammation
pneumoperitonitis
inflammation plus gas
pyoperitonitis
inflammation plus pus

peritoneum inflammation (cont.)
pyopneumoperitonitis
inflammation plus gas and pus
retroperitonitis
inflammation of the retroperitoneal structures
salpingoperitonitis
inflammation of the tubes and peritoneum

peritoneum operation
peritoneotomy

peritoneum shunt
ascites shunt
peritoneovenous shunt
shunting of ascites fluid from the peritoneal cavity to the jugular vein

persecution delusion
paranoia

perspiration
diaphoresis

perspiration deficiency
hyphidrosis
hypohidrosis
olighidria
oligidria

perspiration lacking
adiaphoresis
anhidrosis

perspiration odor
bromhidrosis
bromidrosis
osmidrosis
ozochrotia
denotes foul smelling perspiration

perspiration preventive
adiaphoretic
anhidrotic

perspiration suppression
anhidrosis
ischidrosis

pesthouse
lazaret

pesthouse (cont.)
lazaretto
hospital for treatment of contagious diseases

phagocyte destruction
phagocytolysis
phagolysis

phagocyte enhancer
opsonin
substance in the blood making bacteria more prone to action of phagocytes

phalanges in excess
polyphalangia
polyphalangism

phalanx inflammation
phalangitis

phalanx lacking
hypophalangism
born without one or more bones of finger or toe

phalanx operation
phalangectomy

phalanx shortness
brachyphalangia

pharynx discharge
pharyngorrhea

pharynx disease
pharyngopathy
any abnormal condition of the pharynx

pharynx dryness
pharyngoxerosis

pharynx examination
pharyngoscopy

pharynx inflammation
adenopharyngitis
pharyngotonsillitis
of the pharynx and tonsils
nasopharyngitis
pharyngorhinitis
of the pharynx and nasal passages
pharyngitis
of the pharynx in general

pharynx inflammation (cont.)
pharyngolaryngitis
of the pharynx and larynx
retropharyngitis
of the tissues behind the pharynx
rhinopharyngitis
of the mucous membrane of the nose and pharynx

pharynx obstruction
pharyngemphraxis

pharynx operation
pharyngectomy
pharyngoplasty
pharyngotomy

pharynx pain
pharyngalgia
pharyngodynia

pharynx paralysis
pharyngoparalysis
pharyngoplegia

pharynx spasm
pharyngismus
pharyngospasm

pharynx stone
pharyngolith
calculi of the pharynx
rhinopharyngolith
calculi of the nose and pharynx

pharynx stricture
pharyngoperistole
pharyngostenosis

pharynx viewer
nasopharyngoscope
pharyngoscope
instruments used for examining pharynx and nose

phenetidin in urine
phenetidinuria

phenol poisoning
carbolism

phenol in urine
phenoluria

131

phenyl-ketone in urine
phenylketonuria

phosphates in urine
phosphaturia

phosphorescent sweat
phosphorhidrosis
phosphoridrosis
excretion of luminous sweat

phosphorescent urine
photuria

phosphorus poisoning
phosphorism

phrase repetition
palilalia
paliphrasia
involuntary repetition of words

pigeon breast
pectus carinatum

pigment-lacking disease
achroderma
alphodermia
any disease resulting from lack of pigmentation
achromatosis
albinism
leukoderma
a condition where the skin lacks pigmentation

pigments in urine
acholuria
acholuric
lacking bile pigment in urine
urochrome
uroletin
yellow pigment in urine
urocyanin
uroglaucin
bluish-green pigment in urine
urocyanogen
urocyanosis
blue pigment in urine
urorubin
urofuscohematin

pigments in urine (cont.)
urosein
red pigment in urine
uromelanin
black pigment in urine
urophein
gray pigment in urine
urospectrin
pigment found in normal urine
indican
uroxanthin
yellow pigment that turns indigo blue on oxidation

piles
hemorrhoids

pine-cone shaped
pineal
piniform

pineal gland operation
pinealectomy
removal of the gland

pinkeye
conjunctivitis

pinworm in humans
oxyuriasis

placenta inflammation
placentitis

placenta lacking
aplacental

plant eating
herbivorous
phytophagous
feeds on plants or herbs

plant-fungus disease
schizomycosis
any disease caused by plant microorganisms

plant juice
succus
juice extracted for medicinal purposes

plant life
flora

132

plant poison
phytotoxin
poisonous protein

plantar vesicles
chiropompholyx
dyshidrosis
pompholyx
blisters that appear on the soles of the feet and palms of the hands

plasma separation
plasmapheresis
removal of plasma from withdrawn blood before return to the donor

plasma substitute
periston

plaster
cataplasm
poultice
usually applied to the skin after the plaster has been heated

plastic bone surgery
osteoplasty

plastic cheek surgery
meloplasty

plastic ear surgery
otoplasty

plastic eye surgery
ophthalmoplasty

plastic graft surgery
alloplasty
allotransplantation
transplanted into the same species
autoplasty
transplant from one's own body
heteroplasty
heterotransplantation
transplanted from another species

plastic lip surgery
cheiloplasty
chiloplasty

plastic mouth surgery
stomatoplasty

plastic nose surgery
rhinoplasty

plastic palate surgery
palatoplasty
staphyloplasty
uraniscoplasty
uranoplasty
uranostaphyloplasty
uranostaphylorrhaphy

plastic tissue surgery
zoografting
zooplasty
grafting of animal tissue into the human body

pleasant delusions
habromania
morbid impulse toward gaiety

pleasure diminution
anhedonia

pleura calculus
pleurolith

pleura inflammation
pleurisy
pleuritis
inflammation of the pleura
pleurohepatitis
inflammation of the pleura and liver
pleuropericarditis
inflammation of the pleura and pericardium

pleura operation
pleurectomy
pleuracotomy
pleurotomy
thoracotomy

pleura pain
pleuralgia
pleurodynia

pleural cavity air/gas
pneumothorax

pleural cavity fluid
hydropneumothorax
accumulation of serous fluid and gas

pleural cavity puncture
pleuracentesis
pleurocentesis
thoracentesis

pleural cavity pus
empyema
pyohemothorax
pyopneumothorax
pyothorax

pleurisy/pneumonia
pleuropneumonia

plucking bedclothes
carphology
floccillation
delirious picking during illness considered to be a serious symptom

plucking habit
phaneromania
preoccupation with an external part of the body

plug of cotton
tampon

pneumococci in blood
pneumococcemia

pneumococci in urine
pneumococcusuria

pneumogastric nerve
vagus
nerve located from the cranial cavity to the abdominal organs

pneumonia
pneumonitis
pulmonitis

pneumonia/pleurisy
pleuropneumonia

poem-writing mania
metromania

poikilocytes in blood
poikilocythemia
poikilocytosis
presence of irregularly shaped red blood cells in the peripheral blood

pointed head
acrocephalia
acrocephaly
oxycephaly
turricephaly

poison in blood
septicemia
toxemia
toxicemia

poison fear
toxicophobia
toxiphobia
abnormal fear of poison or being poisoned

poison immunity
mithridatism
immunizing against a poison by gradually increasing the dosage

poison of meat
allantiasis
botulism

poison producing
toxiferous

poison in producing cell
endotoxin
toxin retained in the cell that produces it

polypeptides in blood
polypeptidemia

portal vein dilation
pylephlebectasia
pylephlebectasis

portal vein inflammation
pylephlebitis

portal vein obstruction
pylemphroxis
obstruction of the vein that enters the liver

portal vein relating
pylic

portal vein thrombosis
pylethrombosis

134

postchildbirth discharge
lochia
the mucus, blood and tissue debris discharged after childbirth

postmortem examination
autopsy
necropsy

pot
marijuana

pouch of testicles
scrotum

powerless
adynamia

pregnancy
cyesis

pregnancy classification
multigravida
multipara
pregnant woman who has previously given birth
multiparity
multiparous
polycyesis
having given birth to several children
primigravida
woman pregnant for the first time

pregnancy convulsions
eclampsia

pregnancy diagnosis
cyesiognosis

pregnancy extrauterine
eccyesis
ectopic pregnancy
paracyesis
development of the fertilized ovum outside the cavity of the uterus

pregnancy prevention
contraception

pregnant
gravid

prepuce constricted
phimosis

prepuce inflammation
acroposthitis
posthitis
foreskin

prepuce lacking
aposthia
congenital condition

pressure sense
baresthesia

pressure sore
decubitus ulcer

preventive treatment
chemoprophylaxis
prophylactic
prophylaxis

prism-shaped
prismatic
prismoid

project obsession
zelotypia
compulsive desire for fostering an enterprise

projecting sharp bone
osseous spicule
acidosteophyte*
*obsolete term

projection inflammation
apophysitis
inflammation of the projection of an organ

projection of an organ
apophysis
protruding outgrowth of organ or bone

prone to infectious disease
anaphylaxis
decreased resistance due to effects of previous attacks

prostate discharge
prostatorrhea

prostate inflammation
prostatitis
inflammation of the gland

135

prostate inflammation (cont.)
extraprostatitis
paraprostatitis
periprostatitis
inflammation of the tissues around the gland
prostatovesiculitis
inflammation of the prostate and the seminal vesicles
utriculitis
inflammation of the prostatic utricle

prostate operation
prostatectomy
prostatolithotomy
prostatotomy

protein accumulation
proteinosis
accumulation in the tissues

protein alteration
biotechnology
recombinant protein

protein in blood
carcinoembryonic antigen
proteinemia

protein conversion
proteolysis
conversion into more simple substances

protein, protective
antibody

protein in urine
proteinuria

protoplasm hereditary cells
mitochondria
small specks found in the protoplasm of certain cells

protoxoid of lead
litharge

protozoa-killer
protozoacide

protrusion of cornea
keratectasia

psycho-process measurer
psychodometry
instrument that measures the speed of the psychic process

psychoanalyzed person
analysand

pterygoid canal
Vidian artery
Vidian canal
the internal maxillary artery

puerperal metritis
lochiometritis

pulse clock
sphygmograph
instrument that records pulsation and variations in blood pressure

pulse measurer
pulsimeter
pulsometer
sphygmodynamometer
instrument that measures the force and frequency of the pulse
sphygmochronograph
instrument that registers the pulse related to heart beat

pulse related
sphygmic
sphygmoid

pulse repeated irregularity
allorhythmia
allorhythmic

pulse smallness
microsphygmy
microsphyxia

pulse-wave recorder
kymograph

pulse weakness
acrotism
microsphygmy
microsphyxia
also denotes lack of pulse

puncture with hot needle
ignipuncture

puncture of spine
rachiocentesis

pupil abnormal form
dyscoria

pupil artificial
coremorphosis
formation of an artificial pupil

pupil closure
synizesis

pupil constrictor
miotic

pupil contraction
miosis
mydriatic
myosis*
*obsolete spelling

pupil dilation
corectasia
corectasis
corediastasis
mydriasis
mydriatic

pupil displacement
corectopia

pupil equality
isocoria
two pupils having equal diameter

pupils in excess
polycoria
having more than one pupil in the same orbit

pupil inequality
anisocoria
inequality in diameter

pupils lacking
acorea

pupil measurer
pupillometer
instrument to measure size of the pupil

pupil measurer (cont.)
pupillostatometer
instrument to measure distance between the two pupils
vuerometer
instrument to measure the interpupillary distance

pupil narrowing
stenocoriasis

pupil occlusion
corecleisis
coreclisis

pupil operation
coreoplasty
corepraxy
coreprexy
coroplasty

pupil reflex slow
asthenocoria
slow reaction to a light stimulus

pupil smallness
microcoria

pupil surgical instrument
cortectome

pupillary axis/visual angle
kappa angle

purging
catharsis

purifier
abluent

purines in urine
alloxuria
alloxuric

purple discoloration
livedo reticularis
discoloration of skin caused by dilation of capillaries and venules

purple vision
rhodopsin
erythropsin*
*obsolete term

purpurin in urine
purpurinuria

pus in blood
ichoremia
ichorrhemia

pus containing
purulence
purulency

pus cyst
pyocyst

pus discharge
pyorrhea

pus expectoration
pyoptysis
spitting of pus

pus formation
pyesis
pyogenesis
pyopoiesis
pyosis
suppuration

pus in urine
pyuria

Q

quackery
charlatanism
fraudulent claim to medical knowledge

quartz
silicon dioxide
crystalline form

quicksilver
mercury

quiver
tremor
twitching
involuntary spasmodic movement

R

rabbit eyes
lagophthalmia
lagophthalmos
condition where the eye cannot be
closed entirely

rabbit fever
tularemia

race improvement
euthenics
the science of establishing optimum living conditions

radiant energy measurer
radiomicrometer
detects minute changes in radiant energy
autoradiography
technique to identify tissue binding site

radiant heat, impervious to
adiathermancy

radiant heat measurer
bolometer

radiation therapy
*actinotherapy**
*obsolete term
radiotherapy
sending forth of light, short radio waves,
ultraviolet or x-rays

radioactivity unit
curie
microcurie

rat-bite fever
sodoku

ratlike
murine
also mouse-like

raw flesh eating
omophagia

reaction slow
apathism
delayed response to stimuli

reading impaired
dyslexia

reading slowness
bradylexia

reclining
recumbent

recollection
anamnesis
anamnestic

recovery of strength
analeptic
strengthening, stimulating

rectum examination
proctoscopy
rectoscopy

rectum inflammation
periproctitis
perirectitis
proctitis
rectitis
inflammation of the rectum or anus
coloproctitis
rectocolitis
inflammation of the rectum membrane
and the colon
proctosigmoiditis
inflammation of the rectum and sigmoid
colon

rectum infusion
proctoclysis
through rectal tube

rectum opening to bladder
anus vesicalis
absence of normal opening

rectum operation
proctectomy
proctoplasty
proctotomy
rectectomy
rectoplasty
proctocolpoplasty
proctocystoplasty
proctopexy
rectopexy
proctosigmoidectomy
proctostomy
rectosigmoidectomy
rectostomy
proctotomy
sigmoidoproctostomy

rectum pain
proctagra
proctalgia
proctodynia
rectalgia
pain at the anus or in the rectum

rectum paralysis
proctoparalysis
proctoplegia

rectum prolapse
rectocele
falling of the rectum into the vagina

rectum spasm
proctospasm

rectum specialist
proctologist

rectum stricture
proctostenosis
also called rectostenosis

rectum suture
proctorrhaphy
repair of prolapsed walls

rectum viewer
anoscope
proctoscope
rectoscope
relapse

red blood cell
erythrocyte
reticulocyte

red blood cell clumper
hemagglutinin
a substance

red blood cell formation
erythropoiesis

red corpuscles dissolution
hematolysis
hemolysis
causes failure to coagulate

red discoloration
purpura
purplish or brownish-red discoloration
from hemorrhage into the tissues

red skin patches
erythema

red vision
erythropsia
objects appear to be red

reds
secobarbital
barbiturate

reflex hammer
plessor
plexor
used to test knee reflex

reflex lacking
areflexia

refractive abnormality
ametropia

relapse
palindromia
palindromic

religious insanity
hieromania
belief of inspiration by a divine power

remedy for epilepsy
antiepileptic

remedy for inflammation
antiphlogistic
antipyrotic

remedy for nightmares
antephialtic

remedy for pain
anodyne
analgesic

remedy for scurvy
antiscorbutic

remedy for vomiting
antemetic
antiemetic

remedy for worms
anthelmintic
santonin
vermifuge
used to expel intestinal worms

remote ancestral traits
atavism
characteristics appearing in an individual

renal pelvis dilatation
pyelectasia

renal pelvis operation
pyeloplasty
pyelostomy
pyelotomy
pyelolithotomy

renal pelvis pus
pyonephrosis

repetition
autoecholalia
continuous repetition of one's own
words

reproduction asexual
agamocytogony
agamogony
schizogony

reproductive glands
gonads

resistant to treatment
malignant

respiration
pneusis

respiratory suspension
apnea
apnea vera
when due to decreased carbon dioxide tension
apnea vagal
when due to vagal stimulation

response to contact stimuli
thigmotropism

restlessness
dysphoria

restoration
analeptic
restoring strength

retention in stomach
ischochymia
stagnation of food

retina detachment
amotio retinae

retina examination
retinoscopy
skiascopy

retina image measurer
eikonometer

retina inflammation
retinitis
of the retina
retinochoroiditis
of the choroid and retina
retinopapillitis
of retina and optic disk

retina inner layers
entoretina

retina viewer
retinoscope

rheumatic pain
rheumatalgia

rheumatic study
rheumatology

rhythm defective
dysrhythmia
loss of rhythm, especially an irregularity of heart beat

rhythm lacking
arrhythmia
arrhythmic

rib lacking
apleuria

rib operation
costectomy
costotomy

riblike
costiform

ricelike
riziform

rickets
rachitis
juvenile osteomalacia
in a child

right-eyed
dextrocular
preference in monocular work

right-footed
dextropedal
preference, as in hopping

right-to-left
dextrosinistral

right-side heart
dextrocardia
location on right side

right-twisting
dextrotorsion
as in turning of the eye

ring finger
digitus annularis

ring-shaped
circinate
cricoid

ringing in ears
tinnitus
    sound heard in the ear

ringworm
tinea

r-mispronunciation
rhotacism

rod-shaped
bacilliform
baculiform
rhabdoid

rodent killer
rodenticide

roentgen ray measurer
penetrometer
    instrument to measure the penetrating
    power of an x-ray beam

roof-shaped
tactiform

roof-shaped skull
scaphocephalism
tectocephaly

root operation
radicotomy
rhizotomy

rootlike
rhizoid

ropelike
funic
funicular
    pertaining to the umbilical cord
restiform
    pertaining to nerve fibers

rosalic acid
aurin
corallin
    aromatic dye taken from coal tar

rosin
colophony

rumen inflammation
rumenitis

rumination
merycism
    regurgitation of food

ruminant stomach
1st-rumen
2nd-reticulum
3rd-omasum
4th-abomasum

running ear
otorrhea

running nose
rhinorrhea

rupture
rhexis
    of an organ or vessel

rust of copper
verdigris

S

sac-like
sacciform

sacrum/lumbar vertebra angle
sacrovertebral angle

sacrum operation
sacrectomy
    excision of a segment of the lower verte-
    bral column

sacrum pain
sacralgia
sacrodynia

sacrum proximity
parasacral

St. Vitus dance
ballism
ballismus
chorea
monochorea

saliva
spittle

saliva/air swallowing
aerosialophagy
sialoaerophagy
excessive swallowing of air and saliva in the stomach

saliva deficiency
aptyalia
aptyalism
asialia
hypoptyalism
hyposalivation
xerostomia
deficiency or lack of saliva

saliva duct stricture
sialostenosis

saliva flow excessive
hyperptyalism
hypersalivation
polysialia
ptyalism
ptyalorrhea
salivation
sialism
sialismus
sialorrhea

saliva preventer
antisialagogue
antisialic

saliva promoter
ptyalagogue
sialagogic
sialagogue
a substance that enhances the flow of saliva

saliva suppression
sialoschesis

salivary duct inflammation
sialoangitis
sialodochitis

salivary gland
sialaden

salivary gland inflammation
sialadenitis
sialoadenitis

salivary gland operation
sialoadenectomy
sialoadenotomy
sialithotomy
sialolithotomy
sialodochoplasty

salivation
ptyalism
ptyalosis
sialorrhea
sialosis

salt
saline

salt measurer
salimeter
instrument to measure the amount of salt in solutions

saltlike
haloid

sandfly fever
pappataci fever
phlebotomus fever

sandy
arenaceous
psammous
sabulous

satellite cell
amphicyte

saucerlike
patelliform

scale
squama

scaling horny skin
keratolysis
peeling or scaling off the horny layer on skin

scalp disease
favus
kerion

scalp disease (cont.)
tinea favosa
a type of ringworm usually affecting the scalp

scaly
squamate
squamosa
squamosal
squamous

scaly skin
ichthyosis
pityriasis
a dermatitis marked by scaling

scapula operation
scapulectomy
scapulopexy

scapula pain
scapulalgia
pain in the shoulder blade

scapula pertaining
scapular

scar
cicatrix

scar formation
cicatrization
process of scar formation

scar healing
cicatrize

scar operation
cicatrectomy
cicatricotomy

scar tissue
cheloid
keloid
nodular, lobulated,movable mass of hyperplastic scar tissue

schizophrenia
dementia precox

sciatica
ischialgia
ischiodynia

science of algae
algology
phycology

science of animals
zoology
zoobiology
zoonomy
concerned with the different species of animal life
zootechnics
taming and breeding of animals
zoonosology
zoopathology
classification of diseases of animals

science of arteries
arteriology

science of baths
balneology
science of bathing, as for therapeutic purposes

science of blindness
typhology
study of cause, effects and cure of blindness

science of blood
hematology
hemology

science of blood vessels
angiology
study of blood and lymphatic vessels

science of bones
osteologia
osteology

science of brain
phrenology
an obsolete hypothesis that each form of activity emanates from a separate location in the brain

science of cells
cytology

science of childbirth
obstetrics
tocology

science of children
paidology
pediatrics
pedology

science of climate
climatology
science dealing with climate
phenology
study of climate effect on biological
rhythm of plants and animals

science of deformity
orthopaedics
orthopedics
dealing with prevention and correction of
deformities
teratology
study of congenital malformations and
abnormal development

science of diseases
etiology
term for the cause of disease
pathogenesis
pathogeny
study of origin and development of diseases
pathology
study of cause, symptoms and results of
diseases

science of drugs
pharmacology

science of ears
otiatria
otiatrics
otology

science of ears and throat
otolaryngology

science of ears, nose and throat
otorhinolaryngology

science of excretions
eccrinology

science of eyes
ophthalmology

science of feet
chiropody
podiatry

science of female diseases
gynecology
especially endocrine and reproductive
functions

science of finger signs
cheirology
chirology
dactylology
the art of conveying ideas by means of
the fingers

science of fractures
agmatology

science of fungi
mycology

science of glands
adenology

science of hair
trichology

science of head measuring
cephalometry
science related to measuring the head
or skull

science of heart
cardiology

science of heredity
genetics

science of immunity
immunology

science of inanimate
abiology
anorganology
study of non-living things

science of insects
entomology

science of joints
arthralgia
arthrology
syndesmologia

science of joints (cont.)
syndesmology
synosteology

science of light rays
actinology
radiology

science of limb making
prosthetics
manufacture of artificial parts for the human body

science of liver
hepatology

science of long life
macrobiotics

science of man
anthropogeny
anthropogony
anthropology
study of man's origin and development
somatology
study of the anatomy and physiology of man

science of medicines
pharmacodynamics
study of the effect of medicine on the human body

science of mind
psychology
study of human behavior
psychophysics
study that deals with correlation of mind and matter

science of mouth
stomatology
study of the mouth and its diseases

science of nerves
neurology
study of the nervous system and its disorders

science of nose
rhinology

science of organs
organology
physiology

science of pharynx
pharyngology

science of poisons
toxicology

science of pulse
sphygmology

science of secretions
eccrinology
also applies to excretions
endocrinology
internal secretions

science of sensations
haptics

science of serums
serology
pertaining to antigen and antibody study

science of skin
dermatology

science of stomach
gastrology

science of symptoms
semiology
semiotics
symptomatology

science of treatment
therapeutics
application of remedies for treatment of disease

sclera bulging
sclerectasia
staphyloma
staphylomatous

sclera inflammation
scleritis
sclerotitis
general inflammation
sclerochoroiditis
scleroticochoroiditis
inflammation of the sclera and choroid

sclera knife
sclerotome
surgical instrument for use on the sclera

sclera operation
sclerectomy
scleroplasty
sclerotomy
sclerectoiridectomy
sclerostomy

sclera puncture
scleronyxis

sclera softening
scleromalacia

scoliosis measure
scoliosometry
instrument for measuring the degree of deformity

scotoma measure
scotometry

scraping
abrasion
chemexfoliation
chemical face peeling

scrotal hernia
hydatidocele
orchiocele

scrotum operation
scrotectomy
scrotoplasty

seasickness
naupathia
vomitus marinus

sebaceous cyst
wen

second parturition
secundipara
woman who has borne two children

secretion flow
succorrhea
excessive flow of secretion

secretion high
hypersecretion

secretion low
hyposecretion

secretion of urine
uropoiesis

self-absorption
autism
at the expense of regulation by outward reality
schizophrenia
complex disorder of thinking process and withdrawal

self-analysis
autoanalysis
self-analysis by psychoanalytic method

self-cruelty satisfaction
masochism
finding pleasure in abuses of others

self-hypnotism
autohypnosis
idiohypnotism
self-induced

self-love
autophilia
narcissism

self-starvation
apocarteresis
resulting in death

semen in urine
semenuria
seminuria
spermaturia

seminal deficiency
aspermia
aspermatism

seminal fluid in excess
polyspermia
polyspermism

seminal vesicle inflamed
prostatovesiculitis
vesiculitis

seminal vesicle operation
  vesiculectomy
  vesiculotomy

senile skin
  geroderma
    atrophic skin of the aged

sensation defective
  hypesthesia
  hypoesthesia

sensation lacking
  anesthesia
  dysesthesia

sensitivity to cold
  cryesthesia

sensitivity increased
  anaphylaxis

sensitivity measurer
  baresthesiometer
    instrument to estimate the weight of sensitivity

sensitivity to pain
  algesthesia
  algesia
  algesic
  algetic

septum operation
  septectomy
  septoplasty
  septostomy
  septotomy
    operative procedure on the nasal septum

sequestrum operation
  sequestrectomy
  sequestrotomy

serum study
  serology

severe pain
  megalgia

sex chromosome
  idiochromosome

sexless
  asexual
    having no sex or no sexual interest

sexless reproduction
  agamogenesis

sexual animal attraction
  zoolagnia
    sexual attraction to animals

sexual attraction
  heterosexuality
    for the opposite sex
  homosexuality
    for the same sex

sexual desire
  aphrodisia
  aphrodisiomania
  eroticism
  erotism
  erotomania
  libido
    general terms
  kleptolagnia
    sexual gratification obtained by theft
  necrophilia
  necrophilism
    sexual impulse for contact with dead bodies
  gynecomania
  satyriasis
  satyrism
  satyromania
    strong sexual desire in males
  nymphomania
  nymphomaniac
    strong sexual desire in females
  lesbianism
  sapphism
  tribadism
    homosexuality among females
  pedophilia
    love of children
  pederasty
  sodomy
    anal intercourse
  zooerastia
    attraction to animals

148

sexual desire diminisher
anaphrodisiac
antaphrodisiac
medicinal agent that lessens desire

sexual desire impaired
anaphrodisia

sexual desire promoter
erotic

sexual gratification
autoerotism
autosexualism
masturbation
usually by self-manipulation
algolagnia
increased by inflicting pain
coprolagnia
increased by the thought, sight or handling of feces
masochism
increased by receiving pain from others
psycholagny
increased by mental concepts
pyrolagnia
gratification from setting fires
sadism
gratification from inflicting pain on others
sadomasochism
gratification from either inflicting or receiving pain
iconolagny
induced by sculptures or pictures

sexual impotency
idiogamist
impotent except for one or a few of the opposite sex

sexual intercourse
coitus

sexual perversion
paraphilia
parasexuality

sexual repression
antiorgastic

sexual reproduction
gamogenesis

sexual sensation
hyperhedonia
hyperhedonism

sexually mature
viripotent
obsolete term

shaggy/hairy
hirsute
hirsutism

shaking body
succussion
shaking the body to detect the presence of fluid in the thorax

shapeless
amorphous

sharpness
acuity
acuteness

shaving cramp
xyrospasm

sheath
theca

shedding
exfoliation
detachment of superficial cells from the skin or tissue surface

shin-bone
tibia
the largest bone below the knee

shingles
herpes zoster

shiny skin
leioderma
glossy appearance of the skin

shock therapy
electric shock therapy
electroconvulsive therapy
electroshock therapy
treatment of mental disorder by passage of an electric current through the brain

shortness of breath
dyspnea
   applies to painful and difficult breathing

shortness of fingers
brachydactylia
brachydactyly

shortsightedness
myopia

shoulder blade
scapula

shoulder operation
scapulectomy
scapulopexy

shoulder pain
scapulalgia
scapulodynia

sickle-cell anemia
meniscocytosis

sicklelike
falciform
   shaped like a sickle

side-distortion
rachioscoliosis
scoliosis
   distortion of the spine to one side

sievelike
cribrate
cribriform
polyporous

sigmoid examination
sigmoidoscopy

sigmoid inflammation
sigmoiditis

sigmoid operation
sigmoidectomy
sigmoidotomy
sigmoidopexy
sigmoidoproctostomy
sigmoidorectostomy
sigmoidostomy

sign of death
rhytidosis
   wrinkles of the cornea

signs/gestures lacking
animia
   loss of ability to communicate by gestures

silicon dust disease
anthracosilicosis
   lung disease from inhalation

sinus inflammation
sinuitis
sinusitis

sinus operation
sinuotomy
sinusotomy

sinusitis
aerosinusitis
barosinusitis
   due to difference between internal and external pressures

six children
sextipara
   woman who has borne six children
sextuplet
   one of six children born from the same parturition

six fingers/toes
hexadactylism
hexadactyly

six pregnancies
sextigravida
   pregnant for the sixth time

size cells equal
isocellular

skin aging prematurely
acrogeria
   premature wrinkling and looseness of skin on hands and feet

skin allergic disorder
allergodermia

skin atrophy
atrophia cutis
atrophoderma
atrophodermatosis

skin bleeding
dermatorrhagia
blood discharging from skin

skin blue spot
lividity
black and blue spots on skin

skin bone formation
osteodermia
osteosis cutis

skin color lacking
achromasia

skin cyst
dermatocyst

skin darkening
melanoderma
melasma
due to deposition of excess melanin or
of metallic substances

skin discoloration
dyschroa
dyschroia
poor complexion
chlorosis
chloranemia
chloroanemia
anemic disorder; green sickness
dermatomyositis
purplish red erythema on the face seen
in a progressive muscular disorder

skin disease
dermatopathia
dermatopathy
dermopathy
any disease of the skin
pemphigus
designates a variety of blistering skin
diseases
toxicoderma
toxicodermatosis
disease caused by poison

skin disorder
keratolysis
separation or loosening of the horny
layer of the epidermis
paresthesia
abnormal sensation such as tingling or
burning

skin dryness
fishskin disease
ichthyosis
phrynoderma
xeroderma
xerodermia
xerosis

skin dryness preventer
antixerotic

skin elevation
papule
small, circumcized solid growth
vesicle
containing serum

skin eruption
anthema
generalized, with sudden onset
exanthema
a symptom of an acute viral or coccal
disease

skin glossy and smooth
leiodermia

skin grafting
dermatoplasty
dermoplasty
epidermatoplasty

skin hardening
scleroderma
scleriasis
sclerodermatitis

skin healing imperfect
adermogenesis

skin hemorrhage
petechiasis
formation of minute hemorrhagic spots
in the skin

skin indentation measurer

elastometer
device to measure elasticity of the skin

skin inflammation

acrodermatitis
of the skin of an extremity

dermatitis

scytitis
of the skin in general

eczema
generic term for acute or chronic inflammatory condition of the skin

erysipelas
caused by a hemolytic strep

prurigo
with itching of the papules

pyoderma

pyodermatitis
accompanied by pus

sclerodermatitis
inflammation with hardening

streptodermatitis
due to streptococci

toxicoderma

toxicodermatitis
caused by poison

tungiasis
caused by the gravid sandflea

skin knife

dermatome
used in surgical procedures

skin lacking

adermia

apellous

skin lesion

keratiasis

keratosis
epidermal lesion with circumscribed overgrowths of the horny layer

necrobiosis lipoidica
atrophic shiny lesions on the legs, usually seen in diabetes

skin odor offensive

bromidrosis

ozochrotia

skin ointment

thiol
a mixture of petroleum oils used in treating skin disorders

skin operation

dermatoplasty

skin pain

dermatalgia

dermatodynia

erythromelalgia

rodonalgia

skin parasite

dermatozoan
animal parasite of the skin

skin pigment excessive

hyperchromatism

hyperchromia

skin pigment lacking

achromasia

achromia

achromoderma

leukoderma

leukopathia

leukopathy

skin pinching impulse

dermatothlasia
uncontrollable impulse to pinch and bruise the skin

skin pus disorder

pyoderma

pyodermatitis

pyodermatosis

skin pustules

miliaria pustulosa

periporitis
a form of prickly heat

skin redness

erythema
inflammation due to capillary congestion

skin with scales

ichthyosis

sauriasis

skin sebaceous gland disease
steatoderma
steatosis

skin secretion
seborrhea
stearrhea
steatorrhea
due to indigestion of fat

skin sensitization
photoallergy
photosensitization
sensitivity to light caused by certain drugs or plants

skin smoothness
leiodermia

skin specialist
dermatologist

skin study
dermatology
dermatoglyphics
study of the pattern of ridges of the skin as a genetic indicator

skin swelling
tumefaction

skin thickness
pachyderma
pachydermia
pachydermatosis
pachydermatous
pachyhymenic
pachylosis
pachymenia
tylosis

skin thin/delicate
leptochroa
leptodermic

skin yellow color
xanthochroia
xanthochromia
xanthoderma

skull deformity
scaphocephalism
scaphocephaly

skull with flat vertex
platycephalic
platycephalous
platycephaly

skull inner membrane
endocranium

skull instrument
cranioclast
heavy forceps used to crush head of the fetus
craniotome
surgical instrument used in perforation and crushing of the fetal skull
trephine
instrument used to remove a bone disk from the skull

skull lacking
acrania
acranial
meroacrania
notancephalia
congenital absence of all or part of the cranium

skull measurer
encephalometer

skull operation
craniectomy
cranioclasia
cranioclasis
craniotomy
cranioplasty

skull proportional
orthocephalic
orthocephalous
height in proportion to length and width

skull-sharer
cephalothoracopagus
monocephalus
monocranius
syncephalus
cojoined fetus

skull smallness
leptocephalous
leptocephalus

skull thickness
pachycephalia
pachycephalic
pachycephalous
pachycephaly

sleep abnormal
parahypnosis
as in hypnotism

sleep disorder
central sleep apnea
sleep apnea syndrome
episodes of cessation of breathing during sleep

sleep preventive
antihypnotic

sleep-talking
somniloquence
somniloquism
somniloquist
somniloquy

sleep unnaturally sound
lethargy

sleeping pain
hypnalgia
pain experienced only during sleep

sleeping sickness
encephalitis

sleeplessness
agrypnia
ahypnia
anhypnosis
insomnia

sleepwalking
somnambulance
somnambulism
somnambulist

slightly swollen
tumefaction
tumescence

slimy
glairy
resembling the white of an egg

sling-shaped
fundiform

slit lamp
biomicroscope

smack
heroin

small arms
microbrachia

small body
dwarfism
microsomia
abnormal smallness of the body

small brain convolutions
microgyria

small breasts
micromazia

small calculi
microlith
microlithiasis
a minute calculus consisting of gravel

small chin
microgenia

small colon
microcolon

small cornea
microcornea

small duct
ductule
ductulus
a small tubular structure giving exit to the secretion of a gland

small ears
microtia

small eyeballs
microphthalmia
microphthalmos
microphthalmus
nanophthalmia
nanophthalmos
nanophthalmus
a rare developmental anomaly

small eyelids
microblepharia
microblepharism
microblepharon

small feet
micropodia
micropus

small fingers/toes
micraodactylia
microdactylous
microdactyly

small genital organs
hypogenitalism
microgenitalism

small hands
microcheiria
microchiria
    smallness of the hands

small head
microcephalia
microcephalic
microcephalism
microcephalous
microcephalus
microcephaly

small heart
microcardia
microcardius

small item measurer
acribometer
    instrument for measuring very small objects

small jaw
micrognathia

small lens
microlentia
microphakia
spherophakia
    refers to crystalline lens of the eye

small leukoblast
microleukoblast
micromyeloblast
myeloblast

small lips
microcheilia
microchilia

small mouth
microstomia

small myeloblast
micromyeloblast

small nails
micronychia
    abnormal smallness of the nails

small nipple
microthelia

small penis
micropenis
microphallus

small pupils
microcoria
miosis
    congenital contraction of the pupils

small red blood cells
microerythrocyte
microcyte

small ribbon
teniola

small spinal cord
micromyelia

small stomach
microgastria

small teeth
microdontia
microdontism
microdont
    disproportionate smallness of a tooth or
    teeth to the body build

small tongue
microglossia

small vision
micropsia
    visual disorder causing objects to appear smaller than they are

155

small voice
microphonia
microphony

smallpox
variola
varioloid

smell acuteness
hyperosmia
macrosmatic
oxyosphresia
an exaggerated or abnormally acute sense of smell

smell deficiency
hyposmia
hyposphresia

smell disorder
dysosmia
parasphresia
parosmia
pseudosmia

smell lacking
anodmia
anosmia

smell measurer
olfactometer
device used to measure the keenness of the sense of smell

smell study
osmics
osmology

snake poisoning
ophidiasis
ophidism

sneezing
ptarmus
sternutation

sneeze producer
ptarmic

snow
cocaine

snow blindness
niphablepsia

snow blindness (cont.)
niphotyphlosis
chionablepsia*
*obsolete term

sodium high in blood
hypernatremia
high plasma concentration of sodium ions

sodium low in blood
hyponatremia

sodomy
pederast
pederasty

soft bone tissue
osteogen
tissue that ossifies into bone

soft palate
palatum molle
uvula

soft spot
fontanel
fonticulus
spot in the skull of an infant

softening of...
(see under specific area)

sole
plantar
refers to the sole of the foot

solitude desired
apanthropia
apanthropy

soothing
palliative

sound measurer
phonoautograph
device for recording sound vibrations
phonometer
instrument for measuring the intensity of sound

souring
acescence
ascescent

space
   spatium
   vacuole

Spanish fly
   cantharis
     used as an aphrodisiac

sparseness of hair
   hypotrichiasis
   hypotrichosis
   oligotrichia
   oligotrichosis

sparseness of teeth
   hypodontia
   oligodontia

spasm extending
   protospasm
     spasm that expands to other parts of the body

spasm of fingers
   dactylospasm

spasm-rigidity
   entasis
     rigidity of tonic spasms as in tetanus

speaking fast
   agitolalia
   agitophasia
     excessive rapidity in speech

speaking one word only
   monophasia
     ability to speak only one word or phrase

specks before eyes
   visus muscarum

speech defect
   allophasis
     incoherency
   anaudia
   aphonia
     loss due to injury or disease
   anepia
   aphasia
   aphrasia
     inability to speak

speech defect (cont.)
   amphoriloquy
     speaking with blowing sound
   anarthria
     articulation defective
   aphthongia
     aphasia caused by speech muscles controlled by nerves under the tongue
   apisthyria
     inability to whisper
   bradyarthria
   bradyglossia
   bradylalia
   bradylogia
   bradyphrasia
     slowness in utterance
   cataphasia
     repetition of the same words or phrases
   dyslalia
     due to structural defects of the speech organs or to impaired hearing*dyslogia*
     also impairment of reasoning power
   laloplegia
     inability to speak due to paralysis of muscles
   logopathy
     any speech defect
   mogiphonia
     difficulty due to voice strain
   monophasia
     ability to speak only one word or phrase
   neologism
     use of new and meaningless words
   oxylalia
     speaking with excessive speed
   paralalia
     distortion of sounds
   pyknophrasia
     thickness of speech

speed in speaking
   agitolalia
   agitophasia
   oxylalia

speed in writing
   agitographia
     writing with excessive speed, omitting words or letters

speedball
> *cocaine, heroin*
>> used simultaneously

sperm deficiency
> *oligospermia*
> *oligospermatism*

sperm impotency
> *necrospermia*
>> condition where the sperm are motionless or dead

sperm involuntary loss
> *spermatorrhea*
> *gonacratia**
>> involuntary discharge without orgasm
>> *obsolete term

spermatic duct
> *vas deferens*
>> secretory duct of the testicle

spermatic duct stones
> *spermolith*

sphenoid inflammation
> *sphenoiditis*
>> inflammation of the sphenoid sinus

sphenoid operation
> *sphenoidostomy*
> *sphenoidotomy*

spider bite disorder
> *arachnidism*
> *arachnoidism*
> *araneism*

spider venom antidote
> *antiarachnolysin*

spinal canal open
> *holorachischisis*
> *spina bifida*
>> congenital disorder

spinal column pain
> *rachialgia*
> *rachiodynia*
> *spinalgia*
> *spondylalgia*
> *spondylodynia*

spinal cord
> *medulla spinalis*
> *myelon**
>> *obsolete term

spinal cord defective
> *atelomyelia*

spinal cord disease
> *encephalomyeloradiculopathy*
>> involving the brain, spinal cord and spinal roots
> *myelopathy*
>> any disease of the spinal cord or myeloid tissues
> *myeloradiculopathy*
>> involves spinal cord and nerve roots

spinal cord hemorrhage
> *hematomyelia*
> *myelapoplexy*
> *myelorrhagia*

spinal cord hernia
> *myelocele*
> *myelocystocele*
> *myelomeningocele*
> *meningomyelocele*
> *syringomeningocele*
> *syringomyelocele*
>> defect in closure of the spinal canal with protrusion of cord and membranes

spinal cord inflammation
> *arachnitis*
> *arachnoiditis*
>> of the pia mater and arachnoid
> *cerebrospinal meningitis*
>> of the meninges and spinal cord
> *myelitis*
>> of the bone marrow and spinal cord
> *meningitis*
>> general term
> *meningoencephalomyelitis*
>> of meninges, brain and spinal cord
> *meningomyelitis*
>> of spinal cord and its membranes
> *myeloneuritis*
> *neuromyelitis*
>> multiple neuritis with myelitis

spinal cord inflammation (cont.)

myeloradiculitis
   of the spinal cord and nerve roots
endosteitis
endostitis
perimyelitis
   of the pia mater and spinal cord
polioencephalomeningomyelitis
poliomyelencephalitis
poliomyelitis
   of the gray matter and meninges

spinal cord membrane

meninges
   three membranes enveloping the brain
   and spinal cord
pia mater
   the inner membrane
arachnoid
   the center membrane
dura mater
   the outer membrane

spinal cord smallness

micromyelia

spinal cord softness

myelomalacia

spinal curvature

lordosis
rachioscoliosis
scoliosis

spinal fusion

spondylosyndesis

spinal knife

rachiotome
   surgical instrument used in surgery on
   the vertebrae

spinal matter displacement

heterotopia
   congenital displacement of the gray matter

spinal measurer

rachiometer
   instrument for measuring the degree of
   deformity

spinal nerve inflammation

radiculitis

spinal nerve root disease

radiculopathy

spinal nerve root operation

radiectomy
radicotomy
radiculectomy
rhizotomy

spinal operation

cordotomy
laminectomy
rachiotomy

spinal paralysis

myeloparalysis
myeloplegia
rachioplegia

spinal puncture

rachiocentesis
   surgical procedure

spindle-shaped

fusiform

spineless/headless

acephalorrhachia
   born without head and vertebral column

spinelike

acanthoid
spinous

spiral

helical

spirochete destruction

spirocheticide
spirochetolysis
   destructive to the spirochete bacteria

spirochete disease

spirochetosis

spitting

expectorating

spitting blood

hemoptysis

splanchnic nerve operation
splanchnicectomy
splanchnicotomy
splanchnotomy

spleen
lien
lienal
splenic

spleen disease
splenopathy
lienopathy*
　　*obsolete term

spleen displacement
splenectopia
splenectopy

spleen enlargement
mezalosplenia
splenectasia
splenomegalia
splenomegaly
splenoma
hepatosplenomegaly
splenohepatomegalia
splenohepatomegaly
　　enlargement of both spleen and liver

spleen examination
lienography
splenography

spleen fixation
splenopexia
splenopexy

spleen hernia
lienocele
splenocele

spleen inflammation
splenitis
lienitis*
　　*obsolete term

spleen/kidney
lienorenal
splenonephric
splenorenal

spleen operation
splenectomy
splenopexia
splenopexy
splenotomy

spleen pain
splenalgia
splenodynia

spleen softness
lienomalacia
splenomalacia
splenomyelomalacia
　　of the spleen and bone marrow

spleen suture
splenorrhaphy

spleen tissue destruction
splenolysis

spleen tumor
splenocele
splenoncus

spontaneous generation
abiogenesis
autogenesis

spore largeness
macrospore
megalospore

spot on cornea
albugo
leukoma
　　white spot; cornea opacity

spot/patch
tache

spotted skin
vitiligo
　　white patches
piebaldness
　　different colored patches
livedo
　　black-and-blue spot
xanthoma
　　yellow patches
xanthelasma*
　　*obsolete term

160

sprayer
atomizer
nebulizer
vaporizer

staggering gait
titubation

stagnation in stomach
ischochymia
retention of food

stammering
anarthria
dysarthria
dysphemia
hottentotism
lingual titubation
mogilalia
molilalia
psellism
stammering or stuttering of speech

stapes operation
stapedectomy
stapediotenotomy

star-shaped
asteroid
stella
stellate
stellula

starch
glycogen
animal or liver starch

starch digestion
amylohydrolysis
amylolysis

starch formation
amylogenesis

starch liquefier
galactozymase
a ferment extracted from milk, capable of liquefying starch

starch-sugar conversion
amylolysis

starch in urine
amylosuria
amyluria

starchlike
amylaceous

starchy food undigested
amylodyspepsia
inability to digest

stature shortness
brachymorphic

steal mania
kleptomania
an irrepressible desire to steal

sterility
barrenness
infecundity

sterilization
asexualization
castration
emasculation
tubal ligation
vasectomy

sternum/clavicle
sternoclavicular

sternum fissure
sternoschisis

sternum lacking
asternia
congenital absence of the breast bone

sternum operation
sternotomy

sternum pain
sternalgia
sternodynia

sternum proximity
adsternal
near in location

sticky
viscid

stiffness of joints
ankylosis

stiffness of neck
loxia
torticollis
wryneck

stirrup-bone
stapes
located in the ear

stomach acidity
chlorhydria

stomach dilatation
gastrectasia
gastrectasis

stomach displacement
gastroptosia
gastroptosis
ventroptosia
ventroptosis
downward displacement of the stomach

stomach enlargement
gastromegaly
macrogastria
megastria
megalogastria

stomach hemorrhage
gastrorrhagia

stomach hernia
gastrocele

stomach hormone
gastrin

stomach inflammation
gastritis
the stomach in general
gastradenitis
gastroadenitis
the glands of the stomach
perigastritis
the peritoneal coat of the stomach
enterogastritis
gastroenteritis
gastroenterocolitis
gastroileitis
the stomach and intestine

stomach inflammation (cont.)
gastroesophagitis
the stomach and esophagus
gastroduodenitis
the stomach and duodenum

stomach juice excessive
gastrorrhea

stomach-light
gastrodiaphane
instrument used to illuminate the inside of the stomach

stomach mesentery
mesogaster
mesogastrium

stomach operation
celiogastrostomy
celiogastrotomy
gastrectomy
gastroplasty
gastrostomy
gastrotomy
gastrocolostomy
gastrocolotomy
gastroduodenostomy
gastroenteroanastamosis
gastroenteroplasty
gastroenterostomy
gastrojejunostomy
gastropylorectomy

stomach pain
gastralgia
gastrodynia
peratodynia
stomach ache

stomach secretions
gastroblennorrhea
gastrochronorrhea
gastrohydrorrhea
excessive amounts

stomach smallness
microgastria

stomach spasm
gastrospasm

stomach stapling
gastroplication
gastroptyxis

stomach stone
gastrolith

stomach suture
gastroplication
gastrorrhaphy

stomach viewer
esophagoscope
gastroscope
instrument used for examination

stomach washing
gastrolavage

stone in blood vessel
angiolith
arteriolith
phlebolith

stone breaking
lithodialysis
lithotripsy
crushing or solution of a stone usually in
the bladder or urethra

stone formation
lithiasis
lithogenesis
lithogeny

stone in gallbladder
cholecystolithiasis
cholelithiasis
chololithiasis

stone in lacrimal duct
dacryolith
ophthalmolith

stone passed in urine
lithuresis

stone removal
lithectomy
lithotomy
usually refers to surgical procedure for
urinary stones

stone in ureter
ureterolith

stonecutter disease
silicatosis
silicosis

stonelike
lithoid

strabismus corrector
chiroscope
instrument used for correction

strabismus downward
hypotropia

straightening teeth
orthodontia
orthodontics
branch of dentistry dealing with correction

strain of voice
mogiphonia
difficulty of speech due to voice strain

strength below normal
hyposthenia

strength lacking
adynamia
asthenia
debility

strength measurer
dynamograph
instrument for recording muscular
strength

strengthening
analeptic

stricture cutting
coarctotomy
surgical procedure

stricture of...
(see under specific organ)

striped
striated

strychnine-bearing
ignatia

strychnine-bearing (cont.)
St. Ignatius' bean
strychnos nux vomica

study of...
(see under specific area)

stuttering
lingual titubation
mogilalia
molilalia
stuttering or stammering in general
psellism
due to harelip or cleft palate

sty, stye
hordeolum

subconscious recall
cryptamnesia
cryptomnesia
recalling something previously forgotten

subcostal pain
subcostalgia
pain under the ribs

subnormal temperature
hypothermia

subtongue inflammation
subglossitis
sublinguitis

sucrose in urine
sucrosuria

sudden
fulminant
onset or course of a pain or disorder

suet
sevum

sugar in blood
hyperglycemia
excessive amounts

sugar measurer
saccharimeter
saccharometer

sugar metabolism
saccharometabolism

sugar pill
placebo
inactive substance

sugar in urine
glycosuria
hyperglycosuria
excessive amounts

suicide
apocarteresis
by self-starvation

sun attraction/rejection
heliotaxis
heliotropism
tendency of plants to lean either towards or away from the sun

sun blindness
photoretinitis
photoretinopathy

sun-caused encephalitis
heliencephalitis

sunburn
erythema solare

sunstroke
siriasis
thermoplegia

superior feeling
egomania
extreme self-appreciation

suppression of discharge
ischesis

suppression of sweat
anhidrosis
ischidrosis

suppression of urine
ischuria

suppuration inhibiter
antipyogenic

surgery of abdomen
celiotomy
ventrotomy
opening of the abdominal cavity

surgery of appendix
  appendectomy
  appendicectomy

surgery of arm
  brachiotomy

surgery of bladder
  cystotomy
  lithotomy
  lithotripsy
  lithotrity
  vesicotomy

surgery of bones
  osteorrhaphy
    (see also listings under bones)

surgery of cartilage
  chondrotomy

surgery of cyst
  cystectomy

surgery of fistula
  fistulotomy
  syringotomy
    incision or surgical enlargement of an
    abnormal passage

surgery of gallbladder
  cholecystectomy
  cholecystopexy
  cholecystostomy
  cholecystotomy

surgery of glands
  adenectomy
  adenotomy

surgery of goiter
  strumectomy

surgery of gonad
  gonadectomy
    excision of ovary or testis

surgery of hernia
  celotomy
  herniotomy
  herniorrhaphy
  kelotomy

surgery of joint
  arthrectomy
  arthroplasty
  arthrostomy
  arthrotomy

surgery of kidney
  nephrectomy
  nephrolithotomy
  nephropexy
  nephropyeloplasty
  nephrostomy
  nephrotomy

surgery knife
  bistoury
    small knife used in surgical procedures

surgery of larynx
  laryngectomy
  laryngotomy

surgery needle
  acus

surgery of nerves
  neurectomy
  neuroectomy
  neurotomy

surgery of nympha
  nymphectomy
  nymphotomy
    removal or incision of the labia minora

surgery of ovary
  oophorectomy
  oophorcystectomy
  oophoropexy
  oophoroplasty
  oophorostomy
  oophorotomy
  ovariectomy
  ovariostomy
  ovariotomy

surgery of pancreas
  pancreatectomy
  pancreatoduodenectomy
  pancreatolithectomy
  pancreatolithotomy
  pancreatomy

surgery of pharynx
pharyngectomy
pharyngoplasty
pharyngotomy
procedures involving the portion of the digestive tube between the esophagus and mouth

surgery of sperm duct
vasectomy
for sterilization

surgery of spine
cordotomy
laminectomy
rachiotomy

surgery of spleen
splenectomy
splenopexia
splenopexy
splenorrhaphy
splenotomy

surgery of sterilization
castration
emasculation
spay
tubal ligation
vasectomy

surgery of tendon
tendinoplasty
tendoplasty
tenectomy
tenontoplasty
tenoplasty
tenotomy
procedures involving the fibrous cords or bands connecting muscle to bone

surgery of tongue
glossoplasty
glossotomy

surgery of tonsils
tonsillectomy
tonsillotomy

surgery of tooth
odontectomy
involving excision of surrounding bone

surgery of trachea
tracheoplasty
tracheostomy
tracheotomy

surgery of uvula
staphylectomy
staphyloplasty
staphylotomy
uvulectomy
uvolotomy
usually referring to the uvula attached to the soft palate in the mouth

surgery of veins
phlebectomy
phlebophlebostomy
phleboplasty
phlebotomy
venectomy
venesection
venotomy
venovenostomy

suspended animation
acrotism
asphyxia

suspension of respiration
apnea
temporary absence of breathing

suture of...
(see under specific organ)

swallowing air
aerophagia
aerophagy
pneumophagia

swallowing difficulty
aglutition
aphagia
dysphagia
difficulty or inability to swallow
aphagia algera
due to pain

sweat abnormal
dyshidrosis
dysidria
dysidrosis

sweat in armpits
maschalephidrosis
excessive perspiration

sweat blood
hemathidrosis
hematidrosis

sweat causing
hidrotic
sudorific

sweat deficiency
hyphidrosis
hypohidrosis
olighidria
oligidria

sweat excessive
hyperhidrosis
hyperidrosis
hyperephidrosis
polyhidrosis
polyidrosis
sudoresis

sweat glands
eccrine glands
exocrine glands
small glands covering the entire body

sweat glands inefficient
anaphoresis
anhidrosis
diminished activity

sweat gland inflammation
hidradenitis
hidrosadenitis

sweat odor
bromhidrosis
bromidrosis
osmidrosis
foul smelling perspiration

sweat overflow
hidrosis
sudoresis
profuse sweating

sweat phosphorescent
phosphorhidrosis

sweat preventer
antihydriotic
antisudorific

sweat producing
sudarific
sudoriferous
sudoriparous
carrying or producing sweat

sweat suppression
anhidrosis
hidroschesis
ischidrosis

sweat with urine
urhidrosis
uridrosis
excretion of urea or uric acid in the
sweat

sweeten
edulcorate
to purify from salt, acid or any harsh
substance

sweetener
aspartane
noncaloric substance

swell-producing
tumefacient
tumefy

swelling
tumefaction
tumentia
tumescence

sword-shaped
ensiform
xiphoid

symptomatic hand-writing
macrography
megalographia
large handwriting, usually indicating a
nervous disorder

synovial inflammation
synovitis

synovial operation
synovectomy
villusectomy

synovial tumor
synovioma

syphilitic tumor
gumma
syphiloma
infrequently observed infectuous granuloma characteristic of syphilis

T

tail lacking
acaudal
acaudate

talkativeness
lalorrhea
logorrhea
tachylalia
tachylogia
tachyphasia
tachyphemia
tachyphrasia
usually encountered in individuals with mental disorders

talus operation
astragalectomy

tapeworm
cestoid
cestode
common name for tapeworm

tapeworm disease
teniasis

tapeworm expeller
teniacide
teniafuge

tapeworm head
scolex

tapeworm infestation
cestodiasis

tarsal bone
astragalus
talus
the ankle bone
tarsadenitis
of the tarsal glands and tarsal plate

tarsal operation
tarsectomy
tarsochiloplasty
tarsoplasia
tarsoplasty
tarsotomy

taste abnormal
dysgeusia
abnormality in sense of taste

taste acuteness
hypergeusia
oxygeusia

taste bud
caliculus gustatorius
gustatory bud

taste disorder
parageusia

taste lacking
ageusia
ageustia
loss or impairment of the sense of taste

taste-pertaining
gustatory

taste sense
gustation

taste sense lower
hypogeusia
blunting of the sense of taste

tea drinker
theic

tear flow excessive
dacryorrhea
epiphora

tear gland inflammation
dacryadenitis
dacryoadenitis

tear gland pain
dacryoadenalgia

tear-producer
lacrimator

tear sac
lacrimal sac

tear passage calculus
dacryolith
ophthalmolith
a concretion in the lacrimal apparatus

tear sac inflammation
dacryoblennorrhea
dacryocystoblennorrhea
dacryocystitis

tear sac knife
lacrimotome
surgical instrument

tear sac operation
dacryocystectomy
dacryocystorhinostomy
dacryocystostomy
lacrimotomy

tear sac protrusion
dacryocele
dacryocystocele

teeth...
(see also listings under tooth)

teeth abnormality
odontatrophia
odontatrophy
odontolaxis
odontoloxy
odontoparallaxis

teeth chattering
odonterism

teeth cleaner
odontosmega

teeth deficiency
hypodontia
oligodontia

teeth disease
odontopathy
disease of the teeth or their sockets

teeth in excess
polydentia
polyodontia
presence of supernumerary teeth

teeth extraction
exodontia

teeth fissure
odontoschism

teeth formation
odontogenesis
odontogeny
odontosis

teeth grinding
bruxism
odontoprisis

teeth improper closure
malocclusion

teeth inflammation
odontitis
odontoneuralgia
facial neuralgia caused by tooth decay
parodontitis
peridentitis
periodontitis
of the tissues around a tooth
operculitis
pericoronitis
of the tissues around the crown of a
tooth
pulpitis
of dental pulp

teeth largeness
macrodontia
macrodontism
macrodont

teeth largeness (cont.)
megadont
megalodont

teeth pain
dentalgia
odontalgia
odontodynia
toothache

teeth permanent
monophyodont
having only the permanent set of teeth

teeth similar
homodont

teeth smallness
microdontia
microdontism

teeth straightening
orthodontia
orthodontics
branch of dentistry dealing with correction of irregularities

teeth surgery
odontectomy
odontoplasty
odontotomy

teeth transplanting
allotriodontia
also denotes location of teeth in abnormal places

teeth treatment
dentistry
odontology
odontonosology
odontotherapy

teeth tumor
odontoma

teeth viewer
odontoscope
optical device used in examining teeth

teeth yellow
xanthodont

teething
dentition
odontiasis

tele-influence
automatism
telergy
influence of one individual over the brain of another

temper unrestrained
ecomania
oikomania
particularly in the home environment

temperature elevation
hyperthermia
pyrexia
resulting in fever

temperature evenness
monothermia

temperature measurer
pyrometer
thermometer

temperature subnormal
hypothermia

tendency to murder
hemothymia
a desire to commit murder

tenderness of skin
leptochroa
very thin or delicate skin

tendon fixation
tenodesis

tendon inflammation
peritendinitis
peritenonitis
of tissues surrounding a tendon
thecitis
tenovaginitis
of a tendon sheath
tendosynovitis
tenosynovitis
tendovaginitis
of a tendon and its sheath

tendon knife
tendotome
tenotome
surgical instrument

tendon operation
achillotomy
achillotenotomy
tenectomy
tenodesis
tenonectomy
tenontoplasty
tenoplasty
tenosynovectomy
tenotomy
myotenotomy
tenomyoplasty
tenomyotomy
tenontomyotomy
procedure involving tendon and muscles

tendon pain
tenalgia
tenodynia
tenontodynia

tendon sheath
epitendineum
epitenon
peritenon

tendon suture
tenorrhaphy
tenosuture

tennis elbow
lateral humeral epicondylitis

tension measurer
tensiometer
instrument used to measure the tension of the eyeball, blood vessels, etc.

test tube
in vitro
process or reaction occurring in an artificial environment

terminal proximity
paraterminal

testes in abdomen
cryptorchism
cryptorchidism

testes in excess
polyorchid
polyorchidism
polyorchis
polyorchism
presence of more than two testicles

testes fusion
synorchidism
synorchism
total or partial within the abdomen or scrotum

testis
orchis

testis inflammation
orchiditis
orchitis
orchiepididymitis
epididymo-orchitis

testis operation
cryptorchidectomy
orchidectomy
orchidorrhaphy
orchiectomy
orchiopexy
orchioplasty
orchiotomy
vaso-orchidostomy

testis tumor
orchiocele
sarcocele

tetanic spasm
opisthotonos
opisthotonus
a spasm that bends the body backward

tetanuslike
tetaniform
tetanoid

therapy by air pressure
aerotherapeutics

therapy by animal extract
organotherapy

therapy by baths
balneotherapeutics
balneotherapy
hydrotherapeutics
  treatment by baths and mineral waters

therapy by bone massage
osteopathy

therapy by climate
climatotherapy
  treatment by changing climate

therapy by colored lights
chromophototherapy
chromotherapy

therapy by drugs
pharmacotherapy

therapy by heat
thermotherapy
  treatment by application of heat

therapy by light rays
lucotherapy
phototherapy
  treatment by either solar or artificial light
  rays

therapy by massage
massotherapy

therapy by mechanics
mechanotherapy

therapy by mind
psychotherapeutics
psychotherapy

therapy by nature
naturopathy
  use of natural forces for healing

therapy by opposite
allopathy
heteropathy
  treatment by creating conditions that are
  opposite or different

therapy by radioactivity
radiotherapy
*actinotherapy**
  *obsolete term

therapy by serum
serum therapy

therapy by sun
heliotherapy
  includes sun bathing

therapy by symptom equal
homeopathy
  application of minute doses of an agent
  that would induce similar symptoms in a
  healthy body

therapy by water
balneotherapy
hydrotherapeutics
hydrotherapy
  treatment by external application
thalassotherapy
  treatment by sea-bathing/traveling

thick-fingered
pachydactilia
pachydactylous
pachydactyly

thicken
inspissation
  thickening as by boiling or by evaporation

thickening in excess
pachynis
  abnormal thickening of a part of the
  body

thickening of nails
pachyonychia

thickness of ears
pachyotia

thickness of eyelids
pachyblepharon

thickness of lips
pachycheilia
pachychilia

thickness of skin
pachyderma
pachydermatosis
pachydermia
abnormally thick skin

thickness of skull
pachycephalia
pachycephalic
pachycephalous
pachycephaly

thickness of tongue
macroglossia
pachyglossia

thigh bone
femur
os femoris
the long bone of the thigh

thigh pain
meralgia

thinness of hair
hypotrichiasis
hypotrichosis
oligotrichia
oligotrichosis

thinness of skin
leptochroa
leptodermic
abnormally delicate skin

thirst excessive
anadipsia
hydrodipsomania
polydipsia

thirst lacking
adipsia
adipsy

thoracic fluid
hydrothorax
pleurorrhea
serothorax
accumulation of fluid in the pleural cavity

thorax curved
thoracocyrtosis
abnormally wide curvature of chest wall

thorax/head
cephalothoracic

thorax operation
pleuracotomy
pleurotomy
thoracoplasty
thoracopneumoplasty
thoracostomy
thoracotomy

thorax pain
thoracalgia
thoracodynia

thorax viewer
thoracoscope

thorax/head lacking
acephalothorus
congenital absence

thornlike
acanthoid
spinelike

threadlike
filiform
nematoid
referring to parasitic worms

three-eared
triotus
congenital condition

three-eyed
triophthalmos
congenital condition

three-faced
triopodymus
triprosopus
born with three faces on one head

three-fingered
tridigitate

three-headed
tricephalus
born with three heads

three-ingredient medicine
tripharmacon
tripharmacum

three-layered
trilaminar

three-pointed
tricuspid
tricuspidal
tricuspidate

three testes
triorchism
congenital presence of an additional testis

three-toed
tridigitate

throbbing
palpitation

thrush
apatha
aphthoid
Candida albicans
candidiasis
a thrush fungus

thymus disease
thymopathy
any disease of the small organ located in the lower part of the neck

thymus inflammation
thymitis

thymus operation
thymectomy

thyroid activity increased
hyperthyroidism

thyroid activity normal
euthyroidism

thyroid activity reduced
hypothyroidism
thyroprivia

thyroid hormone excess
thyrotoxicosis

thyroid inflammation
thyroadenitis
thyroiditis

thyroid operation
laryngofissure
thyrochondrotomy
thyrocricotomy
thyroidectomy
thyroidotomy
thyroparathyroidectomy
thyrotomy

thyroid protein
thyroglobulin
thyroprotein
produced by the thyroid gland

tibia pain
tibialgia

tic/spasm
myoclonus multiplex
polyclonia

tic sufferer
tiqueur

tick fever
reovirus infection

tick infestation
ixodiasis

tilting
anteversion
anteverted
condition of being tilted forward
retroversion
retroverted
condition of being tilted backward

time-equal
isochronia
occurring at equal intervals of time

tip-pointed
ensiform
mucronate
xiphoid

tissue change
metaplasia
metaplasis
a change in the structure of adult tissues

tissue clotting
electrocoagulation

tissue destruction
fulguration
by means of a high-frequency electric current

tissue development defective
hypoplasia

tissue dissolution
histolysis

tissue grafting
autograft
heterograft
homograft
isograft
zoograft
zooplasty
grafting of tissues taken from an animal

tissue inflammation
cellulitis
inflammation of the connective tissues
pimelitis
inflammation of adipose or connective tissues
myositis
inflammation of fleshy tissues, as muscle
steatitis
inflammation of adipose tissue

tissue knife
histotome
microtome
surgical instrument

tissue layer
stratum

tissue operation
histotomy
microtomy

tissue separated
slough
necrosed tissue separated from the living structure

tissue study
histologic
histological
histology
histophysiology

tissue with urates
uratosis

tissue with urine
urecchysis

tobacco alkaloid
anatabine
nicotine

toes/fingers abnormally long
arachnodactyly
dolichostenomelia

toes/fingers defective
perodactylia
perodactylus
perodactyly

toes/fingers deficiency
adactylia
adactylism
adactylous
adactyly
oligodactylia
oligodactyly
congenital absence of fingers or toes
monodactylism
presence of only one finger or one toe

toes equal length
isodactylism

toes in excess
hyperdactylia
hyperdactylism
hyperdactyly
polydactyly

toes/fingers fused
syndactylia
syndactylism
syndactylous
syndactylus
syndactyly
zygodactyly

toe inflammation
> *dactylitis*
>> also applies to fingers

toe largeness
> *macrodactylia*
> *macrodactylism*
> *macrodactyly*
> *megadactyly*
> *megalodactyly*
>> also applies to fingers

toe shortness
> *brachydactylia*
> *brachydactyly*
>> also applies to fingers

toe slenderness
> *leptodactylous*
>> also applies to fingers

toe smallness
> *microdactylia*
> *microdactylous*
> *microdactyly*
>> also applies to fingers

toe thickness
> *pachydactylia*
> *pachydactylous*
> *pachydactyly*
>> also applies to fingers

tongue
> *glossa*
> *lingua*

tongue alveolar processes
> *alveolingual*
> *alveololingual*

tongue blackness
> *glossophytia*
> *melanoglossia*

tongue burning
> *glossodynia*
> *glossopyrosis*

tongue/cheeks
> *buccolingual*
>> pertaining to the tongue and cheeks

tongue cyst
> *ranula*
>> cyst under the tongue

tongue disease
> *glossopathy*

tongue displacement
> *glossoptosia*
> *glossoptosis*

tongue with hair
> *glossotrichia*

tongue inflammation
> *glossitis*

tongue inspection
> *glossoscopy*

tongue lacking
> *aglossia*
>> refers to congenital absence and to inability to speak
> *aglossostoma*
>> born without mouth opening

tongue largeness
> *macroglossia*
> *megaloglossia*

tongue membrane
> *periglottis*
>> the mucous membrane of the tongue

tongue operation
> *elinguation*
> *glossectomy*
> *glossoplasty*
> *glossotomy*
> *hemiglossectomy*

tongue pain
> *glossalgia*
> *glossodynia*
> *glossopyrosis*

tongue paralysis
> *glossolysis*
> *glossoplegia*

tongue-pertaining
> *glossal*
> *lingual*

tongue pressure measurer
glossodynamometer

tongue register
glossograph
instrument to measure movements of the tongue

tongue shortness
brachyglossal

tongue smallness
microglossia

tongue spasm
glossospasm

tongue split
schistoglossia

tongue study
glossology

tongue suture
glossorrhaphy

tongue swelling
glossocele
glossoncus
any swelling involving the tongue

tongue thickness
macroglossia
pachyglossia

tongue-tie
ankyloglossia

tonsil inflammation
tonsillitis
adenopharyngitis
pharyngotonsillitis
involving tonsils and pharynx
peritonsillitis
involving tissues surrounding the tonsil

tonsil knife
tonsillotome

tonsil operation
tonsillectomy
tonsillotomy

tonsil stone
tonsillith

tonus lacking
atonia
atonicity
atony

toot
cocaine

tooth...
(see also listings under teeth)

tooth alveolus inflamed
alveolitis

tooth apex locator
apicolocator
instrument used in locating the apex of a tooth

tooth cement in excess
hypercementosis
formation of excessive amount at the root base

tooth deposit
tophus
calcium deposit

tooth disease
odontopathy

tooth disease study
dentistry
odontonosology

tooth hemorrhage
odontorrhagia

tooth operation
apicoectomy
odontectomy
odontoplasty
odontotomy
pulpectomy
pulpotomy
radectomy
*apicectomy**
*obsolete term

tooth pain
odontalgia
odontodynia
toothache

177

tooth probe
tine
pointed tool to explore the tooth

tooth root
apex radicus dentis

tooth sets in excess
polyphyodont
formation of more than two sets of teeth

tooth-shaped
dentiform
dentoid
molariform
odontoid

tooth socket alteration
alveoloplasty
alveoplasty

tooth socket hemorrhage
phatnorrhagia

tooth socket incision
alveolotomy

tooth sparseness
oligodontia
having only a few teeth

tooth splitting
odontoschism

tooth straightener
orthodontist
specialist in aligning teeth

tooth toward cheek
buccoversion
where a tooth extends toward the cheek

tooth treatment
odontotherapy

toothache
aerodontalgia
aero-odontalgia
aero-odontodynia
dentalgia
odontalgia
odontalgic
odontodynia
pulpalgia

toothache reliever
antiodontalgic

toper's nose
rhinophyma

torsion measurer
torsiometer
instrument to measure the ocular torsion

torticollis
loxia
wryneck

touch acuteness
hyperaphia
oxyaphia

touch fear
aphephobia
haphephobia

touch inability
dyscheiria
dyschiria
topagnosis
topoanesthesia
inability to determine site of sensibility

touch measurer
esthesiometer
tactometer
instrument to determine the acuteness
of the sense of touch

touch recognizable
symbolia
ability to recognize an object by touch

touch sense lacking
anaphia
anhaphia
atactilia

touch sensitivity
hyperaphia
oxyaphia
extreme sensitivity to touch

trachea cleft
tracheoschisis

trachea constriction
tracheostenosis

178

trachea hemorrhage
tracheorrhagia

trachea hernia
trachelocele
tracheocele
hernia of the trachea mucous membrane

trachea inflammation
tracheitis
trachitis
tracheobronchitis
tracheopyosis

trachea knife
tracheotome
surgical instrument

trachea operation
tracheoplasty
tracheostomy
tracheotomy

trachea pain
cervicodynia
trachealgia
trachelodynia

trachea pus
tracheopyosis
purulent inflammation

tracing descent
matrilineal
through the female side
patrilineal
through the male side

tranquility
euthymia
mental peace; joyfulness

transformation of tissues
metaplasia
metaplasis
change in structure of adult tissues

transition
metabasis
change in the nature or treatment of a
disease

transposition
metathesis

treatment by...
(see also therapy by...)

treatment by air
aeropiesotherapy
using either compressed or rarified air
aerotherapeutics
aerotherapy
varying pressure or coposition of the air
aerothermotherapy
by means of hot air

treatment by alkali
alkalitherapy

treatment by blood
hematherapy
hemotherapeutics
hemotherapy
transfusion
using blood or blood derivatives for
bleeding disorder or anemia

treatment by causative agent
isopathy

treatment by cold
crymotherapy
cryotherapy

treatment by diet
alimentotherapy

treatment by direct current
galvanotherapy

treatment from distance
teletherapy
administration of x-ray therapy from a
distance

treatment by drugs
chemotherapy
pharmacotherapy

treatment by electric light
electrophototherapy

treatment by electricity
electrotherapeutics
electrotherapy

treatment by fever
pyretotherapy
by induction of fever

treatment by gold
aurotherapy
chrysotherapy
by use of gold compounds

treatment by hypnotism
hypnotherapy

treatment by liver
hepatotherapy
by liver or liver extract

treatment by magnets
magnetotherapy

treatment by massage
massotherapy
naprapathy
reflexotherapy

treatment by milk
galactotherapy
lactotherapy

treatment by movements
kinesiatrics
kinesitherapy

treatment by music
melodiotherapy
musicotherapy

treatment by placenta
placentotherapy
with preparations from animal placentasl

treatment by prayer
theotherapy

treatment by radiation
emanotherapy
radiation therapy
radiotherapeutics
radiotherapy
with x-rays, radium rays or any other radioactive substance

treatment by reduced fluid
dipsotherapy
fluid restriction

treatment by sea
thalassotherapy
by sea travel, sea air or sea baths

treatment by spiritual focus
logotherapy

treatment by vapor
vapotherapy

treatment by vibration
seismotherapy
sismotherapy

treatment by water
hydromassage
hydropathy

treatment by work
ergotherapy
by means of physical exercise

tremor of hands/feet
athetosis
involuntary movements

trench mouth
necrotizing ulcerative gingivitis
also known as Vincent's disease

trichina disease
trichinosis

triple vision
triplopia
single object appears as three

triplet
tridymus

tropical ulcer
phagedena tropica

true ribs
costae verae

trunk lacking
acormus
congenital absence

tube
catheter
salpinx

tube feeding
gastrogavage
gastrostogavage
gavage
providing nourishment through a tube into the stomach

tubes/ovaries inflamed
adnexitis
annexitis

tube pregnancy
salpingocyesis

tuberculosis
consumption
phthisis
obsolete terms

tubular vessel dilatation
ectasia
ectasis
ectatic

tumor
neoplasm
new growth

tumor of blood vessels
angioma

tumor of bone
osteoma
osteophyma
osteophyte

tumor of cartilage
chondroma

tumor cells
oncocytes

tumor of connective tissue
sarcoma
usually highly malignant

tumor destruction
tumoricidal
denoting an agent

tumor dissemination
metastasis

tumor of epithelial cells
carcinoma
epithelioma

tumor of fatty tissue
lipoma

tumor of fibers
fibroma
rhabdomyoma

tumor formation
oncosis

tumor of germ layers
teratoblastoma
teratocarcinoma
teratoma

tumor of glandular tissue
adenocarcinoma
malignant neoplasm
adenoma
usually benign

tumor of jaw
actinomycosis
lumpy jaw

tumor of liver
hepatocarcinoma
hepatoma

tumor of lymph tissue/vessels
angioma
angioma lymphaticum
lymphangioma
lymphoma

tumor of mucous surface
papilloma
villoma

tumor of muscle
myoma
benign neoplasm of muscular tissue

tumor of nerve cells
neuroblastoma

tumor of periosteum
periosteosis
periostosis

tumor of pigment tissue
melanocarcinoma
melanoma

tumor preventor
antineoplastic
preventing development, maturation or spread of neoplastic cells

tumor of striated muscle
rhabdomyoma

tumor of syphilis
gumma
syphiloma

tumor of tendon
tenontophyma
obsolete term

tumor of thyroid
goiter
thyrocele

turbidity measurer
turbidimeter
instrument for determining the degree of cloudiness of a liquid

turpentine poisoning
terebinthism

turpentine tree
terebinth

twin deformities congenital
atlantodidymus
atlodidymus
derodidymus
one body with two heads
cephalothoracopagus
fused head, neck and thorax
craniopagus occipitalis
united at the back of the skull
dicephalus dibrachius
two arms and legs for a double body
dicephalus tetrabrachius
attached from armpits to hips with only two legs
diplopagus
having one or more vital organs in common

twin deformities congenital (cont.)
dipygus parasiticus
omacephalus
pseudoacephalus
thoracoparacephalus
one fetus poorly developed and dependent
ectopagus
ensomphalus
sternopagus
synthorax
thoracopagus
xiphopagus
united at sternal area
ectopagia
ectopagus
thoracopagus
united at the thorax
epigastrius
ilioxiphopagus
omphalopagus
united at the abdomen
epipygus
pygodidymus
pygopagus
united at the buttocks
cephalopagus
iniopagus
united at the back of the neck
metopagus
united at the forehead
monocephalus
monocranius
syncephalus
having one head and two bodies
notomelus
thoracomelus
additional limbs attached to the back or thorax
diprosopus
two faces on a single skull
paragnathus
polygnathus
prosopagus
prosopopagus
attached to the face of the other twin
hemipagus
prosoposternodidymus

twin deformities congenital (cont.)

prosopothoracopagus
united by the face, chest and upper abdomen
rachiopagus
rachipagus
united back to back
somatopagus
having the trunk in common
thoradelphus
attached as one above the umbilicus
triiniodymus
one body with three heads

twisted

tortuous

twisted neck

loxia
torticollis
wryneck

twisting to one side

laterotorsion

twitching

vellication
of the facial muscles
blepharospasm
blepharospasmus
of the eye or eyelid

two-fingered

didactylism
presence of only two digits on a hand or foot

two-formed

dimorphism
dimorphous
existing in two forms

two-headed

atlantodidymus
atlodymus
bicephalous
derodidymus
dicephalus
diplocephalus

two-horned

bicornate
bicornuate
bicornous

two-jawed

dignathus

two-pronged

bifurcate
bifurcated
having two branches

two sets of teeth

diphyodont
normal in humans

tympanic membrane

membrana tympani
myringa

tympanic ring

anulus tympanicus

tympanum inflammation

myringitis
tympanitis
tympanomatoiditis

tympanum operation

myringectomy
myringodectomy
myringoplasty
myringotomy
tympanectomy
tympanotomy

tyrosine in urine

tyrosinuria

U

ulcer

chancre
ulcus
primary lesion of syphilis

ultrasound diagnosis
Doppler echocardiography
sonography
ultrasonography
use of sound to determine location and
measurement of deep structures

umbilical hernia
omphalocele

umbilicus
omphalos

umbilicus bleeding
omphalorrhagia

umbilicus inflammation
omphalitis
omphalophlebitis

umbilicus operation
omphalotomy
omphalotripsy

umbilicus rupture
omphalorrhexis

umbilicus ulceration
omphalelcosis

unborn child
fetus
from the eighth week until the moment
of birth

uncontrollable temper
ecomania
oikomania
noted in the home environment

under tongue
hypoglossal
hypoglossis
hypoglottis
subglossal
sublingual
surface under the tongue

under tongue cyst
ptyalocele
ranula
sialocele
salivary gland cyst

underarm perspiration
maschalyperidrosis
excessive amounts

unhealthful
insalubrious

universal antidote
mithridate
mithridatism
immunity against any poisons

unscaling
desquamation

upper extremities lacking
omacephalus
parasitic twin with imperfect head and
no arms

upper front
anterosuperior
in front and above

upper jawbone
maxilla

upward turning of eyes
anaphoria
anatropia
particularly when at rest

urachus pus
pyourachus

urate deposit
uratosis
in blood or tissues

urates in blood
hyperuricemia
uratemia

urates in urine
uraturia

urea in blood
azotemia
uremia

urea production
Krebs cycle
sequence of chemical reactions in the
liver that produce urea

urea low in urine
hypazoturia
hypoazoturia

ureter calculus
lithureteria
ureterolith
ureterolithiasis

ureter dilation
ureterectasia

ureter disease
ureteropathy
refers to any disease of the ureters

ureter distention
hydroureter
ureterohydronephrosis
uroureter
abnormal distention from accumulation of urine due to obstruction

ureter fistula
ureterostoma

ureter hemorrhage
ureterorrhagia

ureter inflammation
periureteritis
of tissues around the ureter
ureteritis
of the ureter
ureteropyelitis
of ureter and kidney pelvis
ureteropyelonephritis
of ureter, kidney and pelvis
ureteropyosis
accompanied by pus

ureter largeness
megaloureter
megaureter

ureter operation
ureterectomy
ureterolithotomy
ureterolysis
ureteroplasty
ureterostomy
ureterotomy

ureter operation (cont.)
ureteroureterostomy
ureterocolostomy
ureteroenterostomy
ureteroileostomy
ureterosigmoidostomy
involving ureter and intestine
ureterocystostomy
ureteroneocystostomy
ureterovesicostomy
involving ureter and bladder
ureteronephrectomy
ureteropyeloneostomy
ureteropyelonephrostomy
ureteropyelostomy
involving ureter and kidney
ureteroproctostomy
involving ureter and rectum

ureter pain
ureteralgia

ureter pus/mucus
pyoureter
ureterophlegma
ureteropyosis

ureter stricture
ureterostenoma
ureterostenosis

ureter suture
ureterocelorrhaphy
ureterorrhaphy

urethra discharge
urethrorrhea

urethra inflammation
periurethritis
of the tissues connecting the urethra
skeneitis
skenitis
of glands or ducts near the urethra
urethritis
of the urethra itself
urethrocystitis
of the urethra and bladder

urethra knife
urethrotome

urethra opening defective
balanic hypospadias
hypospadiasis
hypospadias perinealis
    congenital defect

urethra operation
urethrectomy
urethroplasty
urethrostomy
urethrotomy

urethra pain
urethralgia
urethrodynia

urethra protrusion
urethrocele
    prolapse of the female urethra

urethra proximity
paraurethral

urethra spasm
urethrism
urethrismus
urethrospasm

urethra stricture
urethrostenosis

urethra suture
urethrorrhaphy

urethra viewer
panendoscope
urethrascope
urethroscope
    instrument for examining the urethra

urethral/anal eroticism
amphimixis
    also signifies union of the chromatins

urethral ring
annulus urethralis
musculus sphincter vesicae

urethral stricture tool
electrolyzer
    instrument for treatment by electrolysis

uric acid disintegration
uricolysis

uric acid excretion
lithuria
uricosuria

urinary canal
ureter
    brings urine from the kidneys to the
    bladder
urethra
    takes urine out of the bladder

urinary nitrogen
azoturia
    excessive amounts

urinary stone expeller
lithagogue

urinate
micturate

urination
emiction
micturition
uresis

urination arrest
anuresis
anuria

urination desire
micturition
    also denotes frequent urination

urination in excess
diuresis
hydruria
polyuria

urination frequency
micturition
nocturia
nycturia
pollakiuria
thamuria

urination impossible
acraturesis
    due to lack of elasticity of the bladder

urination impulse
uresiesthesia
uriesthesia

urination involuntary
   enuresis

incontinence
      usually occurring at night or during sleep

urination pain
   dysuria
   dysury
   urodynia

urine with albumin
   albuminuria
   pseudoalbuminuria

urine with alcohol
   alcoholuria

urine with alkalinity
   alkalinuria
   alkaluria
      the passage of alkaline urine

urine with amebas
   ameburia

urine with amines
   aminuria

urine with amino acids
   acidaminuria
   aminoaciduria
   hyperaminoaciduria

urine with ammonia
   ammoniuria

urine by anus
   urochesia
      passing urine through the anus

urine aromatic odor
   uraroma

urine with bacilli
   bacilluria

urine with bacteria
   bacteriuria
      passage of bacteria in the urine

urine with bile salts
   biliuria
   choleuria
   choluria

urine with bilirubin
   bilirubinuria

urine with black pigment
   melanuria
      excretion of a dark-colored urine

urine with blood
   hematocyturia
   hematuria
   hemuresis

urine with blood/chyle
   hematochyluria
      presence of both in the urine

urine with calcium
   calcariuria
   calciuria
   hypercalciuria
   hypercalcinuria
   hypercalcuria

urine calculus
   urolith
   urolithiasis

urine with carbohydrates
   carbohydraturia

urine with carbolic acid
   carboluria
      presence of phenol in the urine

urine with carbons
   carbonuria

urine with casts
   cylindruria

urine with chlorides
   chloriduria
   chloruresis

urine with cholesterol
   cholesterinuria
   cholesteroluria

urine with chyle or lymph
   chyluria

urine concentrated
   oligohydruria

urine with crystals
crystalluria

urine in a cyst
urinoma
cyst containing urine

urine deficiency
oligohydruria
oliguresia
oliguresis
oliguria

urine with dextrin
dextrinuria

urine with dextrose
glycosuria
glucosuria
dextrosuria*
*obsolete term

urine with diacetic acid
diacetonuria
diaceturia

urine examination
urinalysis
analysis of the components
urinoscopy
uroscopy
by visual observation

urine in excess
polyuria

urine excretion increased
diuresis
diuretic

urine with fat
adiposuria
lipuria
excretion of lipids in the urine

urine with free myoglobin
myoglobinuria

urine with fructose
fructosuria
levelosuria

urine with globulin
globulinuria

urine with gravel
urocheras
uropsammus
any inorganic or uratic sediment in the urine

urine gravity low
hyposthenuria
due to inability of kidneys to concentrate urine

urine gravity measurer
urinometer
urogravimeter
urometer

urine with hematin
urobilin
urofuscohematin
urohematin
urohematoporphyrin
causing presence of red pigment in the urine

urine with hemoglobin
hemoglobinuria

urine with hippuric acid
hippuria
excretion of abnormally large amounts

urine with histidine
histidinuria

urine with histone
histonuria
observed in certain diseases

urine with homogentisic acid
alcaptonuria
alkaptonuria

urine with hyalin
hyalinuria

urine with hydrogen sulfide
hydrothionuria

urine Incontinence
enuresis
occurring usually during sleep

urine with indican
indicanuria

188

urine with indigo
indigouria
indiguria

urine with indole
indoluria

urine with indoleacetic acid
indolaceturia

urine with indoxyl
indoxyluria

urine infiltration
urosepsis
from infiltration of urine into the tissues

urine with inositol
inosituria
inosuria

urine interruptions
urinary stuttering
involuntary jerky urination

urine with ketone
hyperketonuria
ketonuria

urine lacking pigment
acholuria
acholuric

urine with lactose
lactosuria
excretion of milk sugar in the urine

urine with leucine
leucinuria

urine with levulose
levulosuria

urine with lithic acid
hyperlithuria
lithuria

urine with lymph
lymphuria

urine with membrane
meninguria
presence of shreds of membrane in urine

urine with methemoglobin
methemoglobinuria

urine with milkiness
chyluria
galacturia

urine with nitrates
nitrituria

urine with nitrogen
hyperazoturia
presence of excessive amounts

urine nitrogen lacking
anazoturia
also denotes deficiency

urine with oxalic acid
oxaluria
also presence of oxalidates

urine paleness
achromaturia

urine with phenetidin
phenetidinuria

urine with phenols
phenoluria

urine with phenyl-ketone
phenylketonuria

urine with phosphates
phosphaturia
presence of excessive amounts

urine phosphorescent
photuria

urine with protein
proteinuria

urine with purines
alloxuria

urine with purpurin
porphyrinuria

urine with pus
pyuria

urine red
erythruria

urine retention
ischuria
also denotes suppression

urine with saccharose
saccharosuria
obsolete term

urine secretion
uropoiesis
process of urine formation

urine with semen
semenuria
seminuria
spermaturia

urine specific gravity low
hyposthenuria

urine with starch
amyluria

urine with sucrose
sucrosuria

urine sugar
glucosuria
glycosuria
hyperglycosuria
melituria*
*obsolete term

urine sugar lacking
aglycosuria

urine in sweat
urhidrosis
uridrosis
excretion of abnormal quantity of urine
components in sweat

urine in tissues
urecchysis
uredema
uroedema

urine with tyrosine
tyrosinuria

urine with urates
lithuria
uraturia

urine with xanthine
xanthinuria
xanthiuria
xanthuria
presence of excessive amounts

urobilin in blood
urobilinemia

urobilin in urine
urobilinuria

uterus
womb

uterus adhesion
hysterolysis
cutting off the attachment

uterus atony
metratonia
after childbirth

uterus atrophy
metratrophia
metratrophy

uterus closing
hysterocleisis

uterus discharge
lochia
lochial
lochiometra
metrorrhea

uterus disease
hysteropathy
metropathia
metropathy
any disorder of the uterus

uterus displacement
metroptosia
metroptosis
metrectopia*
metrectopy*
*obsolete terms

uterus fibroid operation
fibroidectomy
fibromectomy

190

uterus fixation
hysteropexy
uterofixation
uteropexy

uterus gas distention
physometra

uterus gas/fluid
physohydrometra
accumulation of air and gas

uterus hemorrhage
metrorrhagia
irregular menstrual flow
metrostaxis
slight, persistent flow
metropathia hemorrhagica
abnormal bleeding
polymenorrhea
frequent menstrual periods

uterus hernia
hysterocele

uterus inflammation
metritis
uteritis
of the uterus in general
endometritis
of the inner layer of the uterine wall
metrolymphangitis
of the lymphatic vessels
metroperitonitis
perimetritis
of the uterus and peritoneum
metrophlebitis
of the uterus veins
mesometritis
myometritis
of the muscular tissue
parametritis
of the connecting tissues
perisalpingitis
of the tissues around a tube
pyosalpingitis
pus and inflammation of the uterine tube
pyosalpingo-oophoritis
pus and inflammation of the tube, ovary
and oviduct

uterus inflammation (cont.)
salpingo-oophoritis
of the tubes and ovaries
salpingoperitonitis
of tubes and peritoneum
cervicitis
trachelitis
of the neck of the uterus

uterus lacking
ametria

uterus ligament
ligamentum teres uteri
the round ligament
mesometrium
the wide ligament
mesosalpinx
the upper part of the wide ligament surrounding the tube

uterus measurer
hysterometer
uterometer
instrument for measuring the cavity of
the uterus
metrodynamometer
used to measure contractions
parturiometer
measures expulsive force
uretometer
measures the uterus size

uterus operation
celiohysterectomy
celiohysterotomy
hysterectomy
hysteromyomectomy
hysteromyotomy
hystero-oophorectomy
hysteropexy
metroplasty
metrotomy
hysterosalpingectomy
hysterosalpingo-oophorectomy
hysterotrachelectomy
hysterotrachelotomy
hysterocervicotomy
cervicectomy
cervicotomy

uterus operation (cont.)
trachelectomy
trachelopexia
trachelopexy
tracheloplasty
stomatomy
stomatotomy
    surgical incision to facilitate labor

uterus pain
hysteralgia
hysterodynia
metralgia
metrodynia

uterus paralysis
metroparalysis
    during or after childbirth

uterus pus
pyometra

uterus rupture
hysterorrhexis
metrorrhexis

uterus softness
metromalacia
metromalacoma
metromalacosis
    pathologic softening of the uterine tissues

uterus spasm
uterismus

uterus stone
hysterolith

uterus study
hysterology

uterus suspension
ligamentopexis
ligamentopexy
    shortening of the ligaments

uterus suture
hysterorrhaphy
salpingorrhaphy
trachelorrhaphy

uterus tissues
parametrium
    connective tissues around the uterus

uterus tube cover
perisalpinx

uterus tube gas/pus
physopyosalpinx

uterus tube operation
salpingectomy
salpingoplasty
salpingotomy
tubectomy
salpingo-oophorectomy
salpingoovariectomy
salpingopexy
salpingostomatomy
salpingostomy

uterus tubes and ovaries
adnexa uteri

uterus tumor
hysteromyoma
    benign neoplasm of uterine muscular tissue

uterus varicosity
utero-ovarian varicocele

uterus viewer
hysteroscope
metroscope
uteroscope

utterance slow
bradyarthria
bradyglossia
bradylalia
bradyphasia
    slowness of speech

uvea inflammation
uveitis
uveitic
    of the iris, ciliary body and choroid of the eye

uvula cleft
bifid uvula
staphyloschisis

uvula elongation
staphyloptosis
uvuloptosis

uvula enlargement
staphyledema

uvula inflammation
peristaphylitis
uvulitis

uvula knife
staphylotome
uvulotome
an instrument for cutting the uvula

uvula operation
palatoplasty
staphylectomy
staphyloplasty
staphylotomy
uvulatomy
uvulectomy
uvolotomy

uvula prolapse
staphyloptosis
uvulaptosis
uvuloptosis

uvula suture
palatorrhaphy
staphylorrhaphy
surgical repair of the uvula
palatopharyngorrhaphy
staphylopharyngorrhaphy
surgical repair of the palate and pharynx

vagina atresia
ankylocolpos

vagina contraction
colpospasm

vagina dilatation
colpectasia
colpectasis
distention in general

vagina discharge
lochia
locial
discharge following childbirth

vagina disease
colpopathy
vaginopathy

vagina distention
aerocolpos
caused by gas or air

vagina dryness
colpoxerosis
of the mucous membrane

vagina examination
colpomicroscopy
study of the cells

vagina fluid removal
culdocentesis

vagina fungus disease
colpitis mycotica
colpomycosis
vaginomycosis

vagina gas
flatus vaginalis
expulsion of gas from the vagina

vagina hemorrhage
colporrhagia

agina hernia
colpocele
vaginocele

vagina Inflammation
colpitis
vaginitis
of the vagina in general
pachyvaginitis
with thickening of the walls
paracolpitis
paravaginitis

vagina inflammation (cont.)
pericolpitis
perivaginitis
of the connective tissue around the vagina
colpocystitis
of the vagina and bladder
vulvovaginitis
of the vagina and vulva

vagina laceration
colporrhexis

vagina mucus
hydrocolpocele
hydrocolpos
mucocolpos
accumulation of mucus in the vagina

vagina occlusion
colpatresia
gynatresia

vagina operation
colpectomy
colpocleisis
colpopexy
colpoplasty
colpopoiesis
colpotomy
vaginapexy
vaginectomy
vaginofixation
vaginoplasty
vaginotomy
proctococlytroplasty
proctocolpoplasty
repair of a rectovaginal fistula

vagina pain
colpalgia
colpodynia
vaginism
vaginismus
vaginodynia
vulvismus
spasmodic pain

vagina prolapse
colpoptosia
colpoptosis

vagina proximity
paravaginal

vagina pus
pyocolpos
pyocolpocele

vagina stricture
colpostenosis

vagina suture
colporrhaphy

vagina tissue
paracolpium
the connective tissue

vagina viewer
culdoscope
vaginoscope
instrument for examining the internal
genitalia

valve inflammation
dicliditis
valvulitis

valve knife
valvulotome
surgical instrument

valve operation
valvuloplasty
valvotomy
valvulotomy

vanilla itching
vanillism
skin irritation resulting from contact with
vanilla bean

vaporization
nebulization

variable tension
heterotonia

varicose aneurysm
phlebarteriectasia

varicose inflammation
varicophlebitis
inflammation of a varicose vein

varicose operation
cirsectomy
cirsotomy
varicotomy

varicosity of conjunctiva
varicula
swelling of the veins

vascular system disease
angiopathy

vasomotor disturbance
angioneurosis
vasoneurosis

vein/artery communication
anastamosis

vein congestion
phlebismus

vein dilatation
phelbectasia
varicosis
varix
in general
pylephlebectasia
pylephlebectasis
of the portal vein
phlebismus
due to obstruction

vein displacement
phlebectopia
phlebectopy

vein feeding
phleboclysis
venoclysis
adminsitration of food or drugs

vein hardening
phlebosclerosis
venosclerosis

vein hemorrhage
phleborrhagia

vein inflammation
mesophlebitis
phlebitis
of the middle coat

vein inflammation (cont.)
periangitis
perivasculitis
of the outside coat or tissue
periphlebitis
of the tissues around a vein
peripylephlebitis
pylephlebitis
pylethrombophlebitis
pertaining to the portal vein

vein-nerve network
plexus

vein obstruction
phlebemphraxis
thrombosis of a vein

vein operation
cirsectomy
cirsotomy
phlebectomy
phleboplasty
phlebotomy
phlebophlebostomy
varicocelectomy
varicotomy
venectomy
venesection
venipuncture
venotomy

vein pressure measurer
phlebomanometer

vein rupture
phleborrhexis

vein with salt injection
phleboclysis
injection of saline solution

vein sclerosis
phlebosclerosis
venofibrosis
venosclerosis

vein stone
phlebolite
phlebolith

vein suture
phleborrhaphy

vein twisting
phlebostrepsis
   surgical process

venous/arterial
arteriovenous

vermifuge
anthelmintic
helminthalgogue
helminthic
   used to expel intestinal worms

vertebra column
rachis

vertebra defect
spondylolysis

vertebra disease
rachiopathy
spondylopathy

vertebra inflammation
perispondylitis
   of tissues around the vertebrae
spondylitis
   of the vertebrae
spondylopyosis
   accompanied by pus

vertebra knife
rachiotome
   surgical instrument

vertebra operation
laminectomy
rachiotomy
spondylotomy
vertebrectomy

vertebra pain
spondylalgia

vesical hernia
cystocele

vesical stone crusher
lithoclast
lithotriptor
lithotrite

vesical stone crushing
lithocenosis
litholapaxy
lithotrity
lithotripsy
   surgical procedure involving crushing
   stones in the bladder

vesical stone viewer
cystoscope
lithoscope

vessel displacement
angiectopia
angioplany
   abnormal location

vessel enlargement
angiectasia
angiectasis

vessel inflammation
angiitis
angitis
vasculitis
   of the blood or lymphatic vessels
periangitis
perivasculitis
   of the sheaths and adventitia

vessel measurer
angiometer
   determines vesseldiameter or tension

vessel operation
arteriectomy
phlebectomy
venectomy

vessel plastic surgery
angioplasty

vessel viewer
angioscope

vestibule
utricle
utriculus
   larger membranous sac in the vestibule
   of the labyrinth

vestibule operation
vestibulotomy

vetch/lupine disease
lathyrism
lupinosis
disease caused by eating certain kinds of vetch or pea species

viewer illuminated
celoscope
optical device for illuminating the interior of a cavity

vigorous old age
agerasia

vinegar acid measurer
acetimeter
apparatus to determine content of acetic acid

vinegarlike
acetous

virgin generation
apogamia
apogamy
apomixia
parthenogenesis
nonsexual reproduction

virus in blood stream
viremia

visceral disease virus
cytomegalovirus

viscosity measurer
viscometer
viscosimeter
instrument to determine viscosity of the blood

viscus collapse
splanchnoptosia
splanchnoptosis
visceroptosis

viscus disease
splanchnopathy

viscus displacement
splanchnodiastasis
splanchnectopia

viscus enlargement
organomegaly
splanchnomegaly
visceromegaly

viscus hardening
splanchnosclerosis

viscus hernia
splanchnocele
protrusion of abdominal viscera

viscus inflammation
perivisceritis

viscus knife
viscerotome
surgical instrument used in autopsy

viscus nerve operation
splanchnicectomy
splanchnicotomy
splanchnotomy

viscus pain
visceralgia

viscus smallness
splanchnomicria

viscus stone
splanchnolith
intestinal calculus

vision in darkness
scotopia
also dark adaptation

vision delusion
pseudoblepsia
pseudoblepsis
pseudopsia

vision dimness
amblyopia
amblyopic

vision impaired
dysopia

vision largeness
macropsia
megalopia
megalopsia

vision measurer
campimeter
haploscope
optometer

vision perverted
parablepsia

vision sensitivity
optesthesia

vision smallness
micropsia
objects appear smaller than they are

vision unequal
aniseikonia
antimetropia
images seen differently by the two eyes

visual image distorted
pseudoblepsia
pseudoblepsis
pseudopsia

visual power fatigue
asthenopia
eyestrain

vitamin deficiency
avitaminosis
hypovitaminosis

vitamin intoxication
hypervitaminosis

vitiated appetite
coprophagy
scatophagy
eating of feces
geophagia
geophagism
geophagy
eating earth
pica
craving for unnatural foods

vitreous body inflammation
hyalitis

vitreous body puncture
hyalonyxis

vitreous humor membrane
hyaloid membrane
membrana vitrea
encloses the vitreous humor of the eye

vocal cord inflammation
chorditis
chorditis vocalis

vocal muscle irritability
hyperphonia
overuse of the voice

voice abnormality
paraphonia

voice impairment
dysphonia
difficulty or pain when speaking

voice loss
alalia
anaudia
aphonia

voice roughness
trachyphonia

voice shrillness
oxyphonia
high pitch of voice

voice strain
mogiphonia

voice weakness
hypophonia
leptophonia
microphonia
microphony
phonasthenia

volume measurement
plethysmography
recording of variations in volume of an organ or part

voluntary motion impaired
dyscinesia
dyskinesia

vomit attempt
retching
vomiturition

vomit inducer
emetic
vomitive
vomitory

vomiting
emesis
anticapatory vomiting
associated with chemotherapy

vomiting blood
hematemesis
vomitus cruentus

vomiting caseous matter
caseation
tyremesis
tyrosis

vomiting in excess
hyperemesis

vomiting excrement
copremesis

vomiting pus
pyemesis

voracious appetite
boulimia
bulimia

vulva incision
episiotomy
to facilitate delivery

vulva inflammation
vulvitis
vulvovaginitis

vulva minor lip
nympha

vulva operation
vulvectomy

vulva/perineum suture
episiorrhaphy

vulva surgical incision
episiotomy
perineotomy
performed at childbirth

walking backward
opisthoporeia

walking difficulty
dysbasia

walking inability
abasia
astasia
inability to maintain erect position
astasia-abasia
inability to stand or walk

walking measurer
pedometer
podometer

walking/standing upright
orthograde

wandering
aberrant
erratic

wanderlust
drapetomania
dromomania
poriomania
uncontrollable desire to leave home

wanting to remember
onomatomania
impulse to dwell upon or recall a word or name

warm-blooded
hemathermal
hematothermal
homeothermal
homiothermal
homothermal
refers to animals that are warm-blooded

warm/cold sensation
>*psychroesthesia*
>>experiencing a cold sensation in a warm part of the body

wart
>*thymion*
>*verruca*
>*verruga*

wart-covered
>*verrucose*
>*verrucosis*

wartlike
>*verruciform*

washing out
>*lavage*
>>of a hollow cavity or organ

wasting away
>*atrophic*
>*atrophy*
>>deterioration of flesh and strength

wasting of body
>*kwashiorkor*
>*limophthisis*
>>seen in African children due to starvation
>*marasmic*
>*marasmus*
>*symptosis*
>>due to improper food assimilation
>*bionecrosis*
>*necrobiosis*
>>death of cells

water attraction
>*hydrophilia*
>>tendency of cells and tissues to attract and retain water

water on brain
>*hydrocephalic*
>*hydrocephalus*

water column index
>*hydrospirometer*

water in joints
>*hydrarthrosis*

water in joints (cont.)
>*hydrarthrus*
>*hydrathron*
>>fluid deposit in the cavity of joints

water magnetism
>*hydrotropism*
>>tendency of plants to lean toward or away from a moist surface

water massage
>*hydromassage*

water study
>*limnology*

water treatment
>*aerohydropathy*
>*aerohydrotherapy*
>*affusion*

watery eye
>*epiphora*

watery liquid flow
>*hydrorrhea*

wave-length measurer
>*spectrometer*
>>instrument for measuring wave length of a light ray

weak body
>*hyposthenia*

weak mind
>*deliquescence*
>*deliquium*

weak pulse
>*acrotism*

weak respiration
>*apnea*
>>also absence of breathing

weak voice
>*dysphonia*
>*hypophonia*
>*leptophonia*

weaning
>*ablactation*

webbed digits
syndactyly
most common congenital anomaly of the hand

wedge-shaped
cuneate
cuneiform
sphenoid

wedge-shaped head
sphenocephalus
sphenocephaly

weed
marijuana

weight loss
emaciation
denoting illness

well-being feeling
euphoria
absence of pain or distress

wheat gum
gluten

wheat protein
glutenin

whiskey nose
rhinophyma

white blood cell
leukoblast
leukocyte

white blood cell deficiency
leukopenia

white blood cell destruction
leukocytolysis
leukolysis
disintegration of leukocytes

white blood cell excess
leukocytosis

white blood cell formation
leukocytogenesis
leukopoiesis

white blood cell in urine
leukocyturia

white gangrene
leukonecrosis
gangrene with formation of a white slough

white hair
leukotrichia

white spot on skin
leukoderma
leukopathia
leukopathy

white spot on tongue
leukoplakia
disorder characterized by white spots on the tongue

whitlow
felon
paronychia
inflammation near the nail

whooping cough
pertussis

whorl
verticil

will power impaired/lacking
aboulia
abulia
abulic
dysbulia
inability to make decisions

wind measurer
anemometer
determines velocity

winding
tortuous

windpipe
trachea

windpipe viewer
bronchoscope
also used for obtaining specimens for culture

wine-pertaining
vinic
vinous

wine study
enology

wink
nictate
nictation
nictitation
palpebrate

wisdom expert
megalomania
sophomania
belief in one's supreme knowledge

within the abdomen
intraabdominal

within the artery
intra-arterial

within the atria
intraatrial

within the bladder
intracystic
intravesical
also denotes within a cyst

within blood vessels/lymphatics
intravascular

within the bronchi
endobronchial
intrabronchial

within a cartilage
enchondral
endochondral
intracartilaginous

within a cell
intracellular

within the dura mater
intradural
enclosed by the outer covering of the brain

within the ear
intra-aural

within the eyeball
entoptic
intraocular

within the heart
endocardiac
intracardiac
within one of the chambers of the heart

within a joint
intra-articular

within the liver
intrahepatic

within a lobe/lobule
intralobular
of any organ or structure

within the mouth
intrabuccal
intraoral

within the nasal cavity
intranasal

within a nucleus
intranuclear
of a cell

within the orbit
intraorbital

within the pelvic cavity
intrapelvic

within the peritoneum
intraperitoneal

within the pleural cavity
intrapleural

within the scrotal sac
intrascrotal

within the skin
intracutaneous
intradermal
intradermic
within the substance of the skin

within the skull
intracranial

within the spinal canal
intraspinal

within the spleen
intrasplanic

within the stomach
intragastric

within the trachea
endotracheal

within a tube
intratubal
within any tube

within the urinary bladder
intravesical

within the uterus
intrauterine

within the veins
endovenous
intravenous

within a ventricle
intraventricular
of the brain or heart

without abdominal wall
agenosomus
congenital deformity

without alimentary canal
agastric

without amnion
anamnionic
anamniotic

without anus aperture
aproctia

without appetite
anorexia

without bile pigment
acholuria
acholuric
in the urine

without bile secretion
acholia
acholic

without blood lymphocytes
alymphocytosis
total or partial absence

without brain
pantanencephalia
pantanencephaly
total absence of any part of the brain

without cerebellum
notanencephalia

without cerebrum/cerebellum
anencephalia
anencephaly

without concentration
aprosexia
inability to fix attention on a given subject

without cranial vault
holoacrania

without ear pinnae
anotia
anotus

without epiloon/omentum
anepiploic
lacking the fold of peritoneum passing from the stomach to another abdominal organ

without extremities
acolous
amelia
amelus

without eyes
anophthalmia
anophthalmos
anophthalmus

without face
aprosopia
congenital absence

without feet
apodal
apodia
apodous
apody
apus

without fetus
afetal

without fever
afebrile
apyretic
apyrexia
apyrexial

without fingers
adactylia
adctyly
congenital absence of fingers or toes

without foreskin
apellous
circumsized by surgery
aposthia
congenital absence

without gestures
amimia
loss of ability to communicate by means of gestures or signs

without glands
anadenia
also denotes deficiency

without glomeruli
aglomerular

without hair coloring
canities
gradual dilution of pigment
poliosis
lack of pigmentation

without hands
acheiria
achiria

without intestine
anenterous

without intestinal movement
aperistalsis

without iris
aniridia
irideremia
total or partial absence

without jaws
agnathia
agnathous

without jaws (cont.)
agnathus
absence of jaws
hemignathia
lacking on one side
tocephalus
otocephaly
congenital absence with other deformities

without limbs
lipomeria
absence of one or more

without lips
acheilia
achilia

without lungs
apneumia

without lymph
alymphia
also denotes deficiency

without mammae
amastia
amazia
congenital absence of breasts

without menstruation
amenia
amenorrhea
menostasia
menostasis

without milk
agalactia
agalactosis
agalactous

without mouth
astomia
astomatous
astomous

without mucous secretion
amyxia
amyxorrhea
also denotes deficiency of flow

without muscle formation
amyoplasia

204

without muscle tone
amyotonia
myatonia

without nails
anonychia
anonychosis

without head/neck
atrachelocephalus
congenital absence

without nervous energy
aneuria

without nipples
athelia

without nose
arhinia
arrhinia

without omentum/epiploon
anepiploic

without part of skull
meroacrania

without perception
agnea
auditory agnosia
optic agnosia
tactile agnosia
inability to recognize by the various perceptions

without phalanx
hypophalangism
congenital absence of one or more phalanges

without placenta
aplacental

without prepuce
apellous
circumcised
aposthia
congenital absence

without reflex
areflexia

without rhythm
arrhythmia
arrhythmic

without ribs
apleuria

without sensation
anesthesia
pharmacological or disease-induced

without sense of smell
anosmia
anosmic

without sense of touch
anaphia
anhaphia
atactilia

without signs or gestures
amimia
loss of ability to communicate by signs

without skin
adermia
apellous

without skin pigment
achromoderma
leukoderma

without skull
acrania
acranial
acranius
notancephalia

without sternum
asternia

without strength
adynamia
asthenia
debility

without symptoms
asymptomatic

without tail
acaudal
acaudate

without taste
ageusia
ageustia
loss or impairment of the sense of taste

without teeth
anodontia

without testes
agenitalism
absence of genitals
anorchia
anorchidism
anorchism
absence of testes

without thirst
adipsia
adipsy

without tongue
aglossia
aglossostomia
congenital deformity

without tonus
atonia
atony

without upper extremities
omacephalus
also lacking complete head development

without urinary bladder
acystia

without uterus
ametria

wolf transformation
lycanthropy
insane delusion believing oneself to be a wolf

woman aversion
misogyny

womb
uterus

wood sugar
xylose

wool fat
adeps lanae
used in preparation of ointment

wool grease
suint

woolsorter's disease
anthracemia
pneumanthrax

word-blindness
alexia

word-madness
verbomania
an abnormal flow of speech

word repeating
palilalia
paliphrasia
repetition of words or phrases

worm killer
vermicide
vermifuge

worm vomiting
helminthemesis

wormlike
vermicular
vermiform

wound breathing
traumatopnea
passage of air through a wound in the chest wall

wound fluid
ichor

wound study
traumatology
branch of surgery concerned with injury

woven together
plexus
interlacing network of nerves, blood or lymphatic vessels

wrinkle
ruga

wrinkle operation
rhytidectomy
rhytidoplasty

wrist bone
capitatum
os magnum
the largest of the carpal bones

writer's cramp
cheirospasm
chirospasm
dysgraphia
mogigraphia

writing inability
agraphia
absolute agraphia
acoustic agraphia
amnemonic agraphia
atactic agraphia
literal agraphia
logographia
loss of the ability to write

writing smallness
micrography

writing speed
agitographia
writing with excessive speed, omitting words or letters

wryneck
loxia
torticollis

xanthine in urine
xanthinuria
xanthiuria
xanthuria

xiphoid inflammation
xiphoiditis
inflammation of the xiphoid process of the sternum

x-ray
roentgen

x-ray dermatitis
radiodermatitis

x-ray inflammation
actinoneuritis
radioneuritis
inflammation of the nerves due to x-rays

x-ray measurer
intensimeter
iontoquantimeter
measures intensity or dosage of the x-rays
qualimeter
quantimeter
obsolete devices
radiometer
roentgenometer
measures quality and penetration of the x-rays

x-ray picture
computed tomography scan
radiogram
roentgenogram
planigraphy
planography
tomography
use of a curvilinear motion during x-ray exposure

x-ray specialist
radiologist
roentgenologist

x-ray study
roentgenology

Y

yawning
oscitation

yellow colored
xanthochromatic

yellow jaundice
icteric
icteroid
icterus
yellowish staining of the skin and deeper tissues

yellow nodule
xanthoma
especially of the skin

yellow skinned
xanthochromia
xanthochroous

yellow teeth
xanthodont

yellow vision
xanthopsia
objects appear yellow

yolk deficiency
oligolecithal

yolk in excess
megalecithal

yolk moderate
medialecithal

youthful
ephebic
hebetic
pertaining to youth

EPONYMS

EPONYM	MEDICAL TERM	COMMENT
Aarskog-Scott syndrome	*faciodigitogenital dysplasia*	congenital disorder involving face, scrotum and fingers
Achard-Thiers syndrome	*adrenocortical disorder*	
Addison's disease	*chronic adrenocortical insufficiency*	
Addison-Biermer disease	*pernicious anemia*	
Ahumada-Del Castillo syndrome	*lactation-amenorrhea syndrome*	also known as Argonz-Del Castillo syndrome
Albers-Schonberg disease	*osteopetrosis*	
Albert's disease/syndrome	*hereditary osteodystrophy*	a retrocalcaneal bursitis
Albright's disease	*polyostatic fibrous dysplasia*	
Almeida's disease	*paracoccidiomycosis*	
Alzheimer's disease	*dementia presenilis*	
Andersen's disease	*type 4 glycogenosis*	glycogen storage disease
Apert's syndrome	*type I acrocephalo-syndactyly*	congenital deformity involving cranium and digits
Apert-Crouzon syndrome	*type II acrocephalo-syndactyly*	
Alport syndrome	*progressive nephropathy*	with nerve deafness
Arndt-Gottron syndrome	*scleromyxedema*	
Avelli's syndrome	*jugular foramen syndrome*	unilateral paralysis of the larynx and soft palate

Balint's syndrome	*ocular motor apraxia*	
Bamberger-Marie syndrome	*hypertrophic pulmonary osteoarthropathy*	
Banti's syndrome	*splenic anemia*	chronic congestive enlargement of the spleen
Barrett's syndrome	*chronic peptic ulcer*	of the lower esophagus
Bassen-Kornzweig syndrome	*abetalipoproteinemia*	
Bernard-Sergent syndrome	*acute adrenocortiical insufficiency*	
Bernhardt-Roth syndrome	*meralgia paraesthetica*	tingling, itching and sensation disorder on the outer lower thigh
Besnier-Boeck-Schaumann syndrome	*sarcoidosis*	
Bloch-Sulzberger syndrome	*incontinentia pigmenti*	inherited developmental defect of the skin
Bloom's syndrome	*congenital telangiectatic erythema*	
Boeck's disease	*sarcoidosis*	also known as Schaumann's syndrome
Brissaud-Marie syndrome	*unilateral spasm of tongue and lips*	of hysterical nature
Brugsch's syndrome	*acropachyderma*	
Buerger's disease	*thromboangitis obliterans*	
Burger-Grutz syndrome	*familial hyperlipoproteinemia*	type I
Burnett's syndrome	*milk-alkali syndrome*	
Busse-Buschke disease	*cryptococcus*	yeastlike fungal infection usually affecting the central nervous system
Caffey's syndrome	*infantile cortical hyperostosis*	

Caplan's syndrome	*intrapulmonary nodules*	associated with rheumatoid arthritis and lung disease in coal workers
Carpenter's syndrome	*acrocephalopolysyndactyly*	
Charcot's syndrome	*intermittent claudication*	
Charcot-Weiss-Baker syndrome	*carotid sinus syndrome*	
Cheney syndrome	*acrosteolysis*	with osteoporosis and changes in the skull and jaw
Chotzen syndrome	*acrocephalosyndactyly*	type III
Christ-Siemens syndrome	*anhidrotic ectodermal dysplasia*	
Churg-Strauss syndrome	*allergic granulomatous angiitis*	
Clarke-Hadfield syndrome	*cystic fibrosis of the pancreas*	
Cogan's syndrome	*oculovestibuloauditory syndrome*	abrupt onset of vertigo and tinnitus followed by deafness
Conn's syndrome	*primary aldosteronism*	
Costen's syndrome	*temporomandibular syndrome*	
Crouzon's syndrome	*craniofacial dysostosis*	inherited abnormal structure of the face and skull
Cushing's syndrome	*pituitary basophilism*	
DaCosta's syndrome	*neurocirculatory asthenia*	
Dalrympk's disease	*cyclokeratitis*	inflammation of the ciliary body and cornea
Dandy-Walker syndrome	*congenital hydrocephalus*	
Danielssen's disease	*anesthetic leprosy*	
Darier's disease	*keratosis follicularis*	

213

Darling's disease	*histoplasmosis*	widely distributed infectious disease acquired by inhalation in soil dust
Dego's disease	*epidemia pleurodynia*	also malignant atrophic papulosis
Dejerine's disease	*hereditary hypertrophic neuropathy*	
Dercum's disease	*adiposis dolorosa*	
DeToni-Fanconi syndrome	*cystinosis*	cystine storage disease
Deutschlander's disease	*tumor of metatarsal bone*	
Devic's disease	*neuromyelitis aplasia*	
DiGeorge syndrome	*absence of thymus and parathyroid glands*	
DiGugliemo's syndrome	*acute erythema acute erythremic myelosis*	abnormal growth of tissue in the bone marrow
Donohue's disease	*leprechaunism*	
Down's syndrome	*mongolism*	
Dressler's syndrome	*postmyocardial infarction syndrome*	complications developing several days to weeks following a myocardial infarction
Dubini's disease	*electric chorea*	
Dubin-Johnson syndrome	*chronic idiopathic jaundice*	
Duchenne's disease	*pseudohypertrophic muscular dystrophy progressive bulbar paralysis*	
Duchenne's syndrome	*anterior spinal paralysis with neuritis*	
Duchenne-Aran disease	*progressive muscular atrophy*	

Duhring's disease	*dermatitis herpetiformis*	chronic skin disease with severe itching, vesicles and papules
Duplay's disease	*subacromial bursitis*	
Duroziez' disease	*congenital stenosis of the mitral valve*	
Ebstein's disease	*tricuspid valve displacement*	congenital heart disorder
Ehlers-Danlos syndrome	*cutis hyperelastica*	elastic skin
Ellis-vanCreveld syndrome	*chondroectodermal dysplasia*	
EMG syndrome	*exomphalos, macroglossia, and gigantism*	
Erb's disease	*progressive bulbar paralysis*	involving the muscles of the upper arm
Erb-Charcot disease	*spastic diplegia*	
Erdheim disease	*cystic medial necrosis*	loss of elastic and muscle fibers in the aorta
Eulenburg's disease	*congenital paramyotonia*	
Faber's syndrome	*achlorhydric anemia*	
Fabry's disease	*glycolipid lipidosis*	
Fahr's disease	*progressive calcific deposition*	in the walls of cerebral blood vessels
Fanconi's syndrome	*renal tubular dysfunction*	
Farber's syndrome	*disseminated lipogranulomatosis*	
Feer's disease	*sweating, weakness, and tremor*	also rapid pulse and insomnia
Felty's syndrome	*rheumatoid arthritis*	with splenomegaly and leukopenia
Fenwick's disease	*idiopathic gastric atrophy*	
Fisher's syndrome	*polyneuroradiculitis*	

Folling's disease	*phenylketonuria*	
Forbe's disease	*type 3 glycogenosis*	glycogen storage disease
Fothergill's disease	*trigeminal neuralgia*	
Fournier's disease	*infective gangrene*	involving the scrotum
Foville's syndrome	*hemiplegia*	an alternating type
Fox-Fordyce disease	*apocrine miliaria*	
Franceschetti's syndrome	*mandibulofacial dysostosis*	
Freeman-Sheldon syndrome	*craniocarpotarsal dystrophy*	
Freiberg's disease	*epiphysial ischemic necrosis*	of the second metatarsal head
Gairdner's disease	*angor pectoris*	
Gaisbock's syndrome	*polycythemia hypertonica*	
Gamna's disease	*chronic splenomegaly*	
Gandy-Nanta disease	*siderotic splenomegaly*	
Garre's disease	*sclerosing osteitis*	thickening or increased density of bones
Gaucher's disease	*cerebroside lipoidosis familial splenic anemia*	
Gelineau's syndrome	*familial nonhemolytic jaundice*	
Gerhardt's disease	*erythromelalgia*	throbbing and burning pain in the skin of the legs, feet, and/or hands
Gerlier's disease	*epidemic vertigo*	
German measles	*rubella*	
Gierke's disease	*type 1 glycogenosis*	glycogen storage disorder
Gilbert's disease	*familial nonhemolytic jaundice*	

Gilchrist's disease	*blastomycosis*	
Glanzmann's disease	*thrombasthenia*	
Glanzmann-Riniker syndrome	*x-linked hypogammaglobulinemia*	
Goldenhar's syndrome	*oculoauriculovertebral dysplasia*	
Goldflam disease	*myasthenia gravis*	
Goltz syndrome	*focal dermal hypoplasia*	
Goodpasture's syndrome	*vagal attack*	
Gorham's disease	*disappearing bone disease*	
Gougerot-Blum disease	*pigmented purpuric lichenoid dermatosis*	
Gower's disease	*saltatory spasm*	a type of progressive muscular dystrophy
Gower's syndrome	*vagal attack*	
Graefe's disease	*ophthalmoplegia progressiva*	
Grave's disease	*toxic goiter*	
Greig's syndrome	*ocular hypertelorism*	
Greenfield's disease	*metachromatic leukodystrophy*	one form of an inherited metabolic disorder
Griesinger's disease	*bilious typhoid*	
Grover's disease	*transient acanthoytic dermatosis*	
Gruber's syndrome	*dysencephalia splanchnocystica*	
Guillain-Barre syndrome	*acute idiopathic polyneuritis*	
Gunther's disease	*congenital porphyria*	
GVH disease	*graft versus host disease*	

Hailey-Hailey disease	*familial benign chronic pemphigus*	
Hallopeau's disease	*acrodermatitis continua*	a sterile pustula eruption on the fingers or toes
Hand-Schuller-Christian disease	*generalized lipid histiocytosis of bone*	
Hansen's disease	*leprosy*	
Hashimoto's disease	*lymphadenoid goiter thyroiditis*	
Hayem-Widal syndrome	*icteroanemia*	acquired jaundice destructive to red blood cells
Hebra's disease	*erythema multiforme familial nonhemolytic jaundice*	
Heerfordt's disease	*uveoparotid fever*	
Heine-Medin disease	*acute anterior poliomyelitis*	
Hers' disease	*type 6 glycogenosis*	glycogen storage disease
Heubner's disease	*syphilitic endarteritis obliterans*	of the cerebral vessels
Hirschsprung's disease	*congenital megacolon*	
Hjarre's disease	*coli granuloma*	
Hodgkin's disease	*anemia lymphatica*	also term for lymphoma
Hodgson's disease	*aortic arch dilation*	associated with insufficiency of the aortic valve
Hoppe-Goldflam disease	*myasthenia gravis*	
Huchard's disease	*chronic arterial hypertension*	
Hunt's syndrome	*progressive cerebellar kyphosis*	
Hutchinson-Gilford disease	*progeria*	premature senility syndrome
Hyde's disease	*prurigo nodularis*	

Iceland disease	*epidemic neuromyasthenia*	
Itai-Itai disease	*cadmium poisoning*	a type found in the Japanese
Jadassohn-Lewan-dowsky syndrome	*pachyonychia congenita*	
Jaffe-Lichtenstein disease	*fibrous dysplasia of bone*	
Jaksch's disease	*anemia infantum pseudoleukemica*	
Jansky-Bielschowsky disease	*cerebral sphingolipidosis*	early juvenile type
Jensen's disease	*retinochoroiditis juxtapapillaris*	
Jeune's syndrome	*asphyxiating thoracic dysplasia*	
Jungling's disease	*osteitis tuberculosa*	
Kallmann's syndrome	*hypogonadism with anosmia*	
Kanner's syndrome	*infantile autism*	
Kashin-Bek disease	*osteoarthrosis*	generalized form found in areas of Asia
Katayama syndrome	*schistosomiasis japonicum*	
Kawasaki disease	*mucocutaneous lymph node syndrome*	
Kienbock's disease	*lunatomalacia*	bone destruction following trauma to the wrist
Kimmelstiel-Wilson disease	*glomerulosclerosis*	
Kimura's disease	*angiolymphoid hyperplasia*	with eosinophilia
Klippel's disease	*arthritic general pseudoparalysis*	
Koerber-Salus-Elschnig syndrome	*retraction nystagmus*	

Kohler's disease	*epiphsial aseptic necrosis*	of the tarsal navicular bone or the patella
Kohlmeier-Degos disease	*malignant atrophic papulosis*	
Korsakoff syndrome	*alcohol amnestic disorder*	
Krabbe's disease	*globoid cell leukodystrophy*	
Krause's syndrome	*encephalo-ophthalmic dysplasia*	
Kuf's disease	*cerebral sphingolipidosis*	adult type
Kugelberg-Welander disease	*juvenile muscular atrophy*	
Kussmaul's disease	*polyarteritis nodosa*	inflammation of arteries in the kidney, muscles, heart and gastrointestinal tract
Kyrle's disease	*hyperkeratosis*	
Lafora's disease	*myoclonus epilepsy*	
Lambert-Eaton syndrome	*carcinomatous myopathy*	
Lane's disease	*erythema palmare hereditorium*	inflammatory redness of the skin of the skin of the palms
Laseuque's disease	*mania of persecution*	
Lawrence-Seip syndrome	*lipoatrophy*	
Legg-Calve-Perthes disease	*epiphyseal aseptic necrosis*	of the upper end of the femur
Legionnaire's disease	*Legionella pneumophilia infection*	
Leigh's disease	*necrotizing encephalomyelopathy*	
Leiner's disease	*erythroderma desquamativum*	
Leri-Weill disease	*dyschondrosteosis*	
Leriche's syndrome	*aortoiliac occlusive disease*	

Lermoyez's syndrome	*labyrinthine angiospasm*	
Letterer-Siwe disease	*nonlipid histiocytosis*	
Libman-Sacks syndrome	*nonbacterial endocarditis*	in some cases of disseminated lupus
Lignac-Fanconi syndrome	*cystinosis*	
Lindau's disease	*retinocerebral angiomatosis*	
Little's disease	*spastic diplegia*	
Lobo's disease	*lobomycosis*	a chronic fungal infection of the skin
Loffler's disease	*an endocarditis*	
Loffler's syndrome	*simple pulmonary eosinophilia*	
Lorain's disease	*idiopathic infantilism*	
Lorain-Levi syndrome	*pituitary dwarfism*	
Louis-Bar syndrome	*ataxia telangiectasia*	
Lyell's syndrome	*toxic epidermal necrolysis*	
Lyme disease	*Lyme borreliosis*	
Madelung's disease	*diffuse symmetrical lipomatosis*	
Magitot's disease	*osteoperiostitis*	of the dental alveoli
Maher's disease	*paravaginitis*	
Majocchi's disease	*purpura annularis telangiectodes*	
Malherbe's disease	*pilomatrixoma*	
Manson's disease	*schistosomiasis mansoni*	
Marchiafava-Bignami disease	*corpus collosum degeneration*	seen primarily in chronic alcoholics

Marchiafava-Micheli syndrome	*paroxysmal nocturnal hemoglobinuria*	
Marek's disease	*avian lymphomatosis*	
Marie-Strumpell disease	*ankylosing spondylitis*	
Marion's disease	*posterior urethra obstruction*	congenital disorder
Maroteaux-Lamy syndrome	*mucopolysaccharidosis*	type VI
Martin's disease	*periosteoarthritis*	of the foot
McArdle's disease	*type 5 glycogenosis*	accumulation of glycogen in muscle
Meckel's syndrome	*dysencephalia splanchnocystica*	
Meige's disease	*hereditary lymphedema*	
Melnick-Needles syndrome	*osteodysplasty*	
Menetrier's disease	*hypertrophic gastritis*	
Meniere's disease	*endolymphatic hydrops*	
Merzbacher-Pelizaeus disease	*hereditary cerebral leukodystrophy*	sclerosis of the white matter of the brain
Meyenburg-Altherr-Uehlinger syndrome	*relapsing polychondritis*	also Meyenburg's disease
Meyer's disease	*adenoids*	
Meyer-Betz syndrome	*myoglobinuria*	
Meyer-Schwickerath and Wyers syndrome	*oculodentodigital dysplasia*	
Mibelli's disease	*porokeratosis*	a rare skin disorder
Milian's disease	*ninth-day erythema*	
Milroy's disease	*hereditary lymphedema*	
Milton's disease	*angioneurotic edema*	

Mitchell's disease	*erythromelalgia*	
Mobius disease	*ophthalmoplegic migraine*	
Mondor's disease	*thrombophlebitis of thoracoepigastric vein*	affecting the breast and chest wall
Monge's disease	*chronic mountain sickness*	
Morgagni's disease	*Adams-Stokes syndrome*	
Morquio's syndrome	*mucopolysaccharidosis*	type IV
Morvan's disease	*syringomyelia*	
Moschowitz' disease	*thrombotic thrombocytopenic purpura*	
Mounier-Kuhn syndrome	*tracheobronchomegaly*	enlarged trachea and bronchus
Neftel's disease	*paresthesia of the head and trunk*	
Neumann's disease	*pemphigus vegetans*	development of vegetations on surfaces of ruptured blisters
Nicolas-Favre disease	*lymphogranuloma venereum*	
Niemann-Pick disease	*sphingomyelin lipidosis*	
Norrie's disease	*atrophia bulborum hereditaris*	
Oguchi's disease	*night blindness*	congenital nonprogressive
Ollier's disease	*enchondromatosis*	
Oppenheim's disease	*amyotonia congenita*	
Ormond's disease	*retroperitoneal fibrosis*	idiopathic
Osgood-Schlatter disease	*epiphysial aseptic necrosis*	of the tibial tubercle
Osler's disease	*erythremia* *hereditary hemorrhagic telangiectasia*	

Osler-Vaquez disease	*erythremia*	
Otto's disease	*arthrokatadysis*	
Owren's disease	*parahemophilia*	
Paas' disease	*skeletal deformation*	familial disorder
Paget's disease	*osteitis deformans*	
Panner's disease	*epiphysial aseptic necrosis*	of the humerus
Parkinson's disease	*shaking/trembling palsy*	
Parrot's disease	*pseudoparalysis*	in infants
Pauzat's disease	*osteoplastic periostitis*	of the metatarsal bones
Pavy's disease	*physiologic albuminuria*	cyclic or recurrent
Paxton's disease	*trichomycosis axillaris*	
Pellegrini's disease	*calcific density*	in the medial collateral ligament
Pellizzi's syndrome	*macrogenitosomia precox*	
Pette-Doring disease	*nodular panencephalitis*	
Pfeiffer syndrome	*type V acrocephalo-syndactyly*	congenital deformity of the digits
Pick's disease	*multiple polyserositis*	
Plummer's disease	*hyperthyroidism*	
Plummer-Vinson syndrome	*sideropenic dysphagia*	
Pompe's disease	*type 2 glycogenosis*	accumulation of glycogen in heart, muscle, liver and nervous system
Posadas' disease	*coccidioidomycosis*	
Pott's disease	*tuberculous spondylitis*	
Poulet's disease	*rheumatic osteoperiostitis*	
Pringle's disease	*adenoma sebaceum*	

224

Purtscher's disease	*retinal angiopathy*	caused by trauma
Quincke's disease	*angioneurotic edema*	
Quinguaud's disease	*folliculitis decalvans*	
Rayer's disease	*biliary xanthomatosis*	
Raynaud's disease	*cyanosis of the digits*	idiopathic, paroxysmal, bilateral
Recklinghausen's disease	*neurofibromatosis*	
Recklinghausen's disease of bone	*osteitis fibrosa cystica*	
Refsum's disease	*heredopathia atactica polyneuritiformis*	
Rendu-Osler-Weber disease	*hemorrhagic telangiectasia*	hereditary condition also known as R-O-W syndrome
Reye's syndrome	*post infectuous syndrome*	liver, kidney and brain damage seen in children
Rieger's syndrome	*iridocorneal mesodermal dysgenesis*	
Riga's disease	*frenum erosion*	also ulceration of the tongue
Riley-Day syndrome	*dysautonomia*	familial disorder
Ritter's disease	*toxic epidermal necrolysis*	also term for icterus neonatorum
Robinson's disease	*hidrocystoma*	in the skin of the face
Robles' disease	*ocular onchocerciasis*	
Rokitansky's disease	*acute yellow atrophy of liver*	
Romberg's disease/syndrome	*facial hemiatrophy*	
Rosenbach's disease	*erysipeloid*	also Heberden's nodes
Roth's disease	*meralgia paresthetica*	
Roth-Bernhardt disease	*meralgia paresthetica*	

Rougnon-Heberden disease	*angina pectoris*	
Rust's disease	*spondylarthrocace*	also termed malum vertebrale suboccipitale
St. Vitus dance	*ballism* *ballismus* *chorea* *monochorea*	
Sanfilippo's syndrome	*mucopolysaccharidosis*	
Savill's disease	*dermatitis epidemica*	
Schamberg's disease	*pigmentary dermatosis*	progressive skin disorder
Schaumann's syndrome	*sarcoidosis*	also known as Boeck's disease
Scheie's syndrome	*mucopolysaccharidosis*	type of metabolic disorder
Schenck's disease	*sporotrichosis*	
Scheuermann's disease	*osteochondritis deformans juvenilis dorsi* *epiphysial aseptic necrosis*	of vertebral bodies
Schilder's disease	*encephalitis periaxialis diffusa*	
Scholz' disease	*demyelinating encephalopathy*	familial disorder with loss of myelin sheaths in the brain
Schottmuller's disease	*paratyphoid fever*	
Seabright bantam syndrome	*pseudohypoparathyroidism*	
Senear-Usher disease/syndrome	*pemphigus erythematosus*	
Shaver's disease	*bauxite pneumoconiosis*	
Shy-Drager syndrome	*progressive encephalo-myelopathy*	involving the autonomic nervous system
Simmonds' disease	*hypophysial/pituitary cachexia*	

226

Simon's disease	*progressive lipodystrophy*	defective metabolism of fat
Sneddon-Wilkinson disease	*subcorneal pustular dermatosis*	
Somogyi effect	*reactive hyperglycemia*	followed by hypoglycemia
Spielmeyer-Stock disease	*retinal atrophy*	in amaurotic familial idiocy
Spielmeyer-Vogt disease	*cerebral sphingolipidosis*	late juvenile type
Stargardt's disease	*fundus flavimaculitus*	
Stein-Leventhal syndrome	*polycystic ovary*	
Steinert's disease	*myotonic dystrophy*	
Stevens-Johnson syndrome	*erythema multiforme bullosum/exudativum*	
Sticker's disease	*erythema infectiosum*	
Stickler syndrome	*arthro-ophthalmopathy*	hereditary, progressive
Still's disease	*rheumatoid arthritis*	juvenile type
Strumpell's disease	*spondylitis deformans acute epidemic leuko-encephalitis*	
Strumpell-Marie disease	*ankylosing spondylitis*	
Strumpell-Westphal disease	*pseudosclerosis*	
Sulzberger-Garbe disease	*exudative dermatitis*	discoid and lichenoid types
Sutton's disease	*halo nevus*	
Sweet's disease	*neutrophilic dermatosis*	acute type of skin disorder
Swift's disease	*acrodynia*	
Sylvest's disease	*epidemic pleurodynia*	
Takahara's disease	*acatalasemia*	

227

Takayasu's syndrome	*pulseless disease*	inflammation of the aortic vessels
Talma's disease	*myotonia acquisita*	
Tangier disease	*lipoprotein deficiency*	familial high density type
Tay's disease	*drusen*	
Tay-Sach's disease	*cerebral sphingolipidosis*	infantile type
Taylor's disease	*cutaneous atrophy*	diffuse idiopathic type
Terry's syndrome	*retinopathy*	of prematurity
Thomsen's disease	*myotonia congenita*	
Thorn's syndrome	*salt-losing nephritis*	
Thygeson's disease	*superficial, punctate keratitis*	associated with viral conjunctivitis
Tietze's syndrome	*peristernal perichondritis*	
Treacher Collins' syndrome	*mandibulofacial dysostosis*	
Trousseau's syndrome	*gastric vertigo*	symptomatic of disease of the stomach
Uehlinger's syndrome	*acropachyderma*	
Underwood's disease	*scleremia neonatorum*	
Unna's disease	*seborrheic dermatitis*	
Unverricht's disease	*myoclonus epilepsy*	
Urbach-Wiethe disease	*lipid proteinosis*	
VanBogaert's disease	*inclusion body encephalitis*	
VanBuchem's syndrome	*cortical hyperostosis*	generalized disorder of bone
Vaquez' disease	*erythremia*	
Verner-Morrison syndrome	*pancreatic cholera*	
Vidal's disease	*lichen simplex*	

Vincent's disease	*ulcerative gingivitis*	necrotizing type
Virchow's disease	*congenital encephalitis*	acute type
Vogt syndrome	*double athetosis*	
VonEconomo's disease	*encephalitis lethargica*	
vonGierke's disease	*type 1 glycogenosis*	glycogen accumulation in liver and kidney
vonMeyenburg's disease	*relapsing polychondritis*	
vonRecklinghausen's disease	*neurofibromatosis*	
vonWillebrand's disease	*angiohemophilia hereditary pseudohemophilia*	also referred to as constitutional thrombopathy
Voorhoeve's disease	*osteopathica striata*	
Waardenburg syndrome	*dystopia canthorum*	
Wagner's disease	*hyaloideoretinal degeneration*	inherited disorder of the vitreous body and retina
Wallenberg's syndrome	*posterior inferior cerebellar artery syndrome*	
Wardrop's disease	*onchyia maligna*	
Weber-Christian disease	*nonsuppurative panniculitis*	nodular type
Wegner's disease	*syphilitic osteochrondritis*	
Well's disease	*infectious icterus/jaundice*	
Werdnig-Hoffmann disease	*muscular atrophy*	infantile type
Werlhof's disease	*thrombocytopenic purpura*	idiopathic disorder
Wermer's syndrome	*polyendocrine adenomatosis*	familial type
Wernicke-Korsakoff syndrome	*encephalopathy with psychosis*	associated with chronic alcoholism
Westphal's disease	*pseudosclerosis*	
Weyers-Thier syndrome	*oculovertebral dysplasia*	

Whipple's disease	*intestinal lipodystrophy*	
Whytt's disease	*internal hydrocephalus*	
Wilkie's disease	*superior mesenteric artery syndrome*	
Wilson's disease/syndrome	*hepatolenticular degeneration*	also exfoliative dermatitis
Winiwarter-Buerger disease	*thromboangitis obliterans*	
Winkelman's disease	*pallidal degeneration*	inherited progressive disorder
Winkler's disease	*chondrodermatitis*	
Wohlfart-Kugelberg-Welander disease	*juvenile muscular atrophy*	
Ziehen-Oppenheim disease	*dystonia musculorum deformans*	progressive torsion spasm of childhood

COMMON MEDICAL ABBREVIATIONS

A	alive; ambulatory; apical; artery; assessment
A2	aortic second sound
AA	amino acid; achievement age; active assistance; arm ankle (pulse ratio); authorized absence; auto accident
AAA	abdominal aortic aneurysmectomy/aneurysm
AAC	antibiotic agent-associated colitis
AAL	anterior axillary line
AAN	analgesic-associated nephropathy; analgesic abuse nephropathy; attending's admission notes
AAO x 3	awake and oriented to time, place and person
AAP	assessment adjustment pass
AAPC	antibiotic acquired pseudomembranous colitis
AAROM	active assistive range of motion
AAS	atlantoaxis subluxation
AAV	adeno-associated virus
AAVV	accumulated alveolar ventilatory volume
Ab	abortion; antibody
A & B	apnea and bradycardia
ABC	airway, breathing, circulation; absolute band counts; artificial beta cells
ABCDE	botulism toxoid pentavalent
Abd	abdomen; abdominal
ABDCT	atrial bolus dynamic computer tomography
ABE	acute bacterial endocarditis
ABG	arterial blood gases
ABI	atherothrombotic brain infarction
ABL	allograft bound lymphocytes
ABLB	alternate binaural loudness balance
ABMT	autologous bone marrow transplantation

ABN	abnormality
abnor.	abnormal
ABR	absolute bed rest; auditory brain (evoked) responses
ABS	at bedside; admitting blood sugar; absorption
ABT	aminopyrine breath test
ABW	actual body weight
ABx	antibiotics
AC	acute; before meals; acromio-clavicular; air conduction; air conditioned; assist control; abdominal circumference; anchored catheter
A/C	anterior chamber (of the eye)
ACA	anterior cerebral artery; acrodermatitis chronicum atrophicans; acute or chronic alcoholism
ACB	antibody-coated bacteria
AC & BC	air and bone conduction
ACBE	air contrast barium enema
ACC	accommodation; adenoid cystic carcinomas; administrative control center
ACD	anterior chest diameter; anterior chamber diameter; anemia of chronic disease; absolute cardiac dullness
ACEI	angiotensin-converting enzyme inhibitor
ACH	adrenal cortical hormone
ACI	aftercare instructions
ACL	anterior cruciate ligament
ACLS	advanced cardiac life support
ACPP-PF	acid phosphatase prostatic fluid
ACT	activated clotting time; allergen challenge test
Act Ex	active exercise
ACTSEB	anterior chamber tube shunt encircling band
ACV	atrial/carotid/ventricular

AD	Alzheimer's disease; right ear; accident dispensary	**AGA**	acute gonococcal arthritis; appropriate for gestational age
ADAU	adolescent drug abuse unit	**AGD**	agar gel diffusion
ADCC	antibody-dependent cellular cytotoxicity	**AGE**	angle of greatest extension
		AGF	angle of greatest flexion
ADD	attention deficit disorder; adduction	**AGG**	agammaglobulinemia
		aggl.	agglutination
ADDU	alcohol and drug dependence unit	**AGL**	acute granulocytic leukemia
ADEM	acute disseminating encephalomyelitis	**AGN**	acute glomerulonephritis
		AGPT	agar-gel precipitation test
ADH	antidiuretic hormone	**AGS**	adrenogenital syndrome
ADL	activities of daily living	**AHA**	autoimmune hemolytic anemia
ad lib	as desired; at liberty	**AHC**	acute hemorrhagic conjunctivitis; acute hemorrhagic cystitis
ADM	admission		
adol	adolescent		
ADPKD	autosomal dominant polycystic kidney	**AHD**	autoimmune hemolytic disease
		AHF	antihemophilic factor
ADR	adverse drug reaction; acute dystonic reaction	**AHG**	antihemophilic globulin
		AHM	ambulatory Holter monitoring
ADP	adenosine diphosphate	**AHT**	autoantibodies to human thyroglobulin
ADS	anonymous donor's sperm; anatomical dead space		
		AI	aortic insufficiency; artificial insemination; allergy index
ADT	anticipate discharge tomorrow		
ADX	adrenalectomy	**A & I**	Allergy and Immunology department
AE	above elbow; air entry		
AEC	at earliest convenience	**AI-Ab**	anti-insulin antibody
AED	automated external defibrillator	**AICA**	anterior inferior communicating artery; anterior inferior cerebellar artery
AEG	air encephalogram		
AER	acoustic evoked response; auditory evoked response		
		AICD	automatic implantable cardioverter/defibrillator
Aer. M	aerosol mask		
Aer. T	aerosol tent	**AID**	artificial insemination donor; automatic implantable defibrillator
AES	anti-embolic stocking		
AF	atrial fibrillation; acid-fast; amniotic fluid; anterior fontanel		
		AIDS	acquired immune deficiency syndrome
AFB	acid-fast bacilli; aorto-femoral bypass	**AIE**	acute inclusion body encephalitis
		AIF	aortic-iliac-femoral
AFC	air filled cushions	**AIH**	artificial insemination with husband's sperm
A.fib	atrial fibrillation		
AFO	ankle-foot orthosis		
AFP	alpha-fetoprotein	**AIHA**	autoimmune hemolytic anemia
AFV	amniotic fluid volume	**AILD**	angioimmunoblastic lymphadenopathy
AFVSS	afebrile, vital signs stable		
A/G	albumin to globulin ratio	**AIMS**	abnormal involuntary movement scale
Ag	antigen		
AG	anti-gravity; anion gap	**AIN**	acute interstitial nephritis

AINS	anti-inflammatory non-steroidal	**AMegL**	acute megokaryoblastic leukemia
AION	anterior ischemic optic neuropathy	**AMG**	acoustic myography
AIP	acute intermittent porphyria	**AMI**	acute myocardial infarction
AIR	accelerate idioventricular rhythm	**AML**	acute myelogenous leukemia
AIVR	accelerated idioventricular rhythm	**AMM**	agnogenic myeloid metaplasia
		AMMOL	acute myelomonoblastic leukemia
AJ	ankle jerk	**amnio**	amniocentesis
AK	above knee	**AMOL**	acute monoblastic leukemia
AKA	above knee amputation; alcoholic ketoacidosis; all known allergies	**AMP**	amputation; ampule
		A-M pr	Austin-Moore prosthesis
ALAT	alanine transaminase (alanine aminotransferase; SGPT)	**AMR**	alternating motor rates
		AMS	acute mountain sickness; amylase
Alb	albumin	**AMV**	assisted mechanical ventilation
ALC	acute lethal catatonia; alcohol	**AMSIT**	A-appearance; M-mood; S-sensorium; I-intelligence; T-thought process (portion of the mental status examination)
ALC R	alcohol rub		
ALD	alcoholic liver disease; adrenoleukodystrophy		
ALDOST	aldosterone		
ALFT	abnormal liver function tests	**amt**	amount
ALG	antilymphocyte globulin	**AMY**	amylase
alk	alkaline	**ANA**	antinuclear antibody;
ALK-P	alkaline phosphatase	**ANAD**	anorexia nervosa and associated disorders
ALL	acute lymphocytic leukemia		
ALM	acral lentiginous melanoma	**ANC**	absolute neutrophil count
ALMI	anterolateral myocardial infarction	**AND**	anterior nasal discharge
		anes	anesthesia
ALP	alkaline phosphatase	**ANF**	antinuclear factor; atrial natriuretic factor
ALS	amyotrophic lateral sclerosis; acute lateral sclerosis; advanced life support		
		ANG	angiogram
		ANLL	acute nonlymphoblastic leukemia
ALT	alanine aminotransferase (SGPT); Argon laser trabeculoplasty	**ANOVA**	analysis of variance
		ANP	atrial natriuretic peptide
ALWMI	anterolateral wall myocardial infarct	**ANS**	autonomic nervous system; answer
AM	myopic astigmatism; amalgam; morning	**ant**	anterior
		ante	before
AMA	against medical advice; antimitochondrial antibody	**A & O**	alert and oriented
		AOAP	as often as possible
AMAP	as much as possible	**AOB**	alcohol on breath
A-MAT	amorphous material	**ao-Il**	aorta-iliac
Amb	ambulate; ambulatory	**AOC**	area of concern
AMC	arm muscle circumference	**AODM**	adult onset diabetes mellitus
AMD	age-related macular degeneration	**AOM**	acute otitis media
		AOP	aortic pressure

A&O x 3	awake and oriented to person, place, and time	**ARF**	acute renal failure; acute rheumatic fever; acute respiratory failure
A&O x 4	awake and oriented to person, place, time and date	**ARLD**	alcohol related liver disease
AOSD	adult onset Still's disease	**ARM**	artificial rupture of membranes
A & P	auscultation and percussion; anterior and posterior; assessment and plans	**AROM**	active range of motion; artificial rupture of membranes
		ARS	antirabies serum
AP	anterior-posterior; antepartum; apical pulse; abdominal-peritoneal; appendicitis	**ART**	arterial; automated reagin test (for syphilis)
		ARV	AIDS related virus
		AS	aortic stenosis; arteriosclerosis; anal sphincter; left ear; activated sleep; ankylosing spondylitis
A2>P2	second aortic sound greater than second pulmonic sound		
APB	atrial premature beat; abductor pollicis brevis	**ASA I**	healthy patient with localized pathological process
APC	atrial premature contraction	**ASA II**	patient with mild to moderate systemic disease
APCD	adult polycystic disease		
APD	automated peritoneal dialysis; atrial premature depolarization	**ASA III**	patient with severe systemic disease limiting activity but not incapacitating
APE	acute psychotic episode		
APKD	adult onset polycystic kidney disease	**ASA IV**	patient with incapacitating systemic disease
APL	acute promyelocytic leukemia; abductor pollicis longus; accelerated painless labor; chorionic gonadotropin	**ASA V**	moribund patient not expected to live (American Society of Anesthesiologist classifications)
appr	approximate	**ASAA**	acquired severe aplastic anemia
appt	appointment		
APR	abdominoperineal resection	**ASAP**	as soon as possible
APTT	activated partial thromboplastin time	**ASAT**	aspartate transaminase (aspartate aminotransferase) (SGOT)
AQ	achievement quotient		
aq	water	**ASB**	anesthesia standby; asymptomatic bacteriuria
aq dist	distilled water		
AR	aortic regurgitation	**ASC**	altered state of consciousness; ambulatory surgery center
A & R	advised and released		
A-R	apical-radial (pulse)	**ASCVD**	arteriosclerotic cardiovascular disease
ARB	any reliable brand		
ARC	AIDS related complex; anomalous retinal correspondence	**ASD**	atrial septal defect
		ASE	acute stress erosion
		ASH	asymmetric septal hypertrophy
ARD	adult respiratory distress; acute respiratory disease; antibiotic removal device	**ASHD**	arteriosclerotic heart disease
		ASIS	anterior superior iliac spine
		AsM	myopic astigmatism
ARDS	adult respiratory distress syndrome	**ASMI**	anteroseptal myocardial infarction

236

ASO	antistreptolysin-O titer; arteriosclerosis obliterans
ASOT	antistreptolysin-O titer
ASP	acute suppurative parotitis
ASS	anterior superior supine
AST	aspartate aminotransferase; astigmatism
ASTZ	antistreptozyme test
ASU	acute stroke unit
ASVD	arteriosclerotic vessel disease
AT	applanation tonometry; atraumatic; antithrombin
ATB	antibiotic
ATC	around the clock
ATD	autoimmune thyroid disease; antithyroid drug
AtFib	atrial fibrillation
ATG	antithymocyte globulin
ATHR	angina threshold heart rate
ATL	Achilles tendon lengthening; atypical lymphocytes; adult T-call leukemia
ATLS	advanced trauma life support
ATN	acute tubular necrosis
ATNC	atraumatic normocephalic
aTNM	autopsy staging of cancer
ATNR	asymmetrical tonic neck reflux
ATPS	ambient temperature and pressure; saturated with water vapor
ATR	Achilles tendon reflex; atrial
ATT	arginine tolerance test
AU	allergenic units; both ears
AUC	area under the curve
AV	arteriovenous; atrioventricular; auditory-visual
AVA	arteriovenous anastomosis
AVD	apparent volume of distribution
AVF	arteriovenous fistula
AVH	acute viral hepatitis
AVM	atriovenous malformation
AVN	atrioventricular node; arteriovenous nicking; avascular necrosis
AVR	aortic valve replacement
AVS	atriovenous shunt
AVSS	afebrile, vital signs stable
AVT	atypical ventricular tachycardia

A&W	alive and well
A waves	atrial contraction waves
AWI	anterior wall infarct
AWOL	absent without leave
ax	axillary
A-Z test	Ascheim-Zondek test; diagnostic test for pregnancy
B	bacillus; bands; bloody; black; both; buccal
Ba	barium
BA	backache; bile acid; blood alcohol; Bourns assist
BAC	blood alcohol concentration; buccoaxiocervical
BAD	bipolar affective disorder
BaE	barium enema
BAE	bronchial artery embolization
BAEP	brain stem auditory evoked potential
BAER	brain stem auditory evoked response
BAL	blood alcohol level; bronchoalveolar lavage
BAO	basal acid output
BAP	blood agar plate
baso.	basophil
BAVP	balloon aortic valvuloplasty
BB	bed bath; bowel or bladder; breakthrough bleeding; blood bank; blow bottle
BBA	born before arrival
BBB	bundle branch block; blood brain barrier
BBBB	bilateral bundle branch block
BBD	benign breast disease
BBM	banked breast milk
BBS	bilateral breath sounds
BBT	basal body temperature
BBVM	brush border vesicle membrane
BC	birth control; blood culture; Bourn control; bed and chair
BCA	balloon catheter angioplasty; basal cell atypia; brachiocephalic artery
BCAA	branched-chain amino acids
BCC	basal cell carcinoma

BCD	basal cell dysplasia
BCE	basal cell epithelioma
B cell	large lymphocyte
BCG	bacillus Calmette-Guerin vaccine
BCL	basic cycle length
BCP	birth control pills
BCS	battered child syndrome; Budd-Chiari syndrome
BD	birth defect; brain dead; bronchial drainage
BDAE	Boston Diagnostic Aphasia Examination
BDI SF	Beck's Depression Index-Short Form
BDR	background diabetic retinopathy
BE	barium enema; below elbow; bacterial endocarditis; base excess; bread equivalent
BEAM	brain electrical activity mapping
BEC	baterial endocarditis
BEE	basal energy expenditure
BEI	butanol-extractable iodine
BEP	brain stem evoked potentials
BF	black female
BFP	biologic false positive
BFT	bentonite flocculation test
BFUE	erythroid burst-forming unit
BG	blood glucose
BGC	basal ganglion calcification
BGM	blood glucose monitoring
BHI	biosynthetic human insulin
BHN	bridging hepatic necrosis
BHS	beta-hemolytic streptococci
BI	bladder irritation; bowel impaction
BIB	brought in by
BID	twice daily
BIG 6	analysis of 6 serum components
BIH	bilateral inguinal hernia; benign intracranial hypertension
bil	bilateral
BILAT SLC	bilateral short leg cast
BILAT SXO	bilateral salpingo-oophorectomy
bili	bilirubin
BILI-C	conjugated bilirubin
BIMA	bilateral internal mammary arteries
BIW	twice a week
BJ	bone and joint
BJE	bones, joints, and examination
BJM	bones, joints, and muscles
BJ protein	Bence-Jones protein
BK	below knee
BKA	below knee amputation
Bkg	background
BLB	Boothby-Lovelace-Bulbulian (oxygen mask)
bl cult	blood culture
BLE	both lower extremities
BLESS	bath, laxative, enema, shampoo and shower
BLOBS	bladder obstruction
BLS	basic life support
B.L. unit	Bessey-Lowry unit
BM	basal metabolism; black male; bone marrow; bowel movement; breast milk
BMA	bone marrow aspirate
BMC	bone marrow cells
BMI	body mass index
BMJ	bones, muscles, joints
BMR	basal metabolic rate
BMT	bone marrow transplant; bilateral myringotomy tubes
BMTU	bone marrow transplant unit
BNO	bladder neck obstruction
BNR	bladder neck retraction
BO	body odor; bowel obstruction; behavior objective
BOA	born on arrival; born out of asepsis
BOM	bilateral otitis media
BOO	bladder outlet obstruction
BOT	base of tongue
BOW	bag of water
BP	blood pressure; bed pan; British Pharmacopeia
BPD	biparietal diameter; bronchopulmonary dysplasia

BPF	bronchopleural fistula	BU	Bodansky unit
BPG	bypass graft	BUE	both upper extremities
BPH	benign prostatic hypertrophy	BUN	blood urea nitrogen
BPM	breaths per minute; beats per minute	BUR	back-up rate (ventilator)
BPRS	Brief Psychiatric Rate Scale	BUS	Bartholin, urethral and Skene's glands
BPSD	bronchopulmonary segmental drainage	BVL	bilateral vas ligation
BPV	benign paroxysmal vertigo	BW	birth weight; body weight; body water
Bq	becquerel	BWCS	bagged white cell study
BR	bathroom; bedrest; Benzing retrograde	BWFI	bacteriostatic water for injection
BRAO	branch retinal artery occlusion	BWS	battered woman syndrome
BRATT	bananas, rice, applesauce, tea and toast	Bx	biopsy
BRB	blood-retinal barrier	C	carbohydrate; Celsius; hundred; cyanosis; clubbing
BRBPR	bright red blood per rectum		
BRJ	brachial radialis jerk	C1	first cervical vertebra
BRM	biological response modifiers	C1 to C9	precursor molecules of the complement system
BRP	bathroom privileges		
BS	blood sugar; bowel sounds; breath sounds; bedside; before sleep	C-II	controlled substance, class 2
		CA	cardiac arrest; carcinoma; carotid artery; chronologic age; coronary artery
B & S	Bartholin and Skene (glands)		
BSA	body surface area	C & A	Clinitest and Acetest
BSB	body surface burned	CAA	crystalline amino acids
BSC	bedside commode	CAB	coronary artery bypass
BSE	breast self examination	CABG	coronary artery bypass graft
BSER	brain stem evoked responses	CaBI	calcium bone index
BSGA	beta Streptococcus group A	CABS	coronary artery bypass surgery
BSO	bilateral salpingo-oophorectomy	CACI	computer assisted continuous infusion
BSOM	bilateral serous otitis media	CAD	coronary artery disease
BSPM	body surface potential mapping	CAE	cellulose acetate electrophoresis
BSS	balanced salt solution; black silk sutures	CAFT	Clinitron® air fluidized therapy
BSU	Bartholin, Skene's, urethra	CAH	chronic active hepatitis; chronic aggressive hepatitis; congenital adrenal hyperplasia
BT	bladder tumor; brain tumor; breast tumor; blood transfusion; bedtime; bituberous		
		CAL	calories; callus; chronic airflow limitation
BTB	break-through bleeding	CALD	chronic active liver disease
BTFS	breast tumor frozen section	CALGB	Cancer and Leukemia Group B
BTL	bilateral tubal ligation	CALLA	common acute lymphoblastic leukemia antigen
BTPS	body temperature pressure saturated		
		CAN	cord around neck
BTR	bladder tumor recheck	CAO	chronic airway obstruction

CAP	capsule; compound action potentials
CAPD	chronic/continuous ambulatory peritoneal dialysis
CAR	cardiac ambulation routine
CARB	carbohydrate
CAS	carotid artery stenosis
CAT	computed axial tomography; children's apperception test; cataract
cath	catheter; catheterization
CAVB	complete atrioventricular block
CAVC	common arterioventricular canal
CAVH	continuous arteriovenous hemofiltration
CB	code blue; chronic bronchitis; cesarean birth; chair and bed
C & B	crown and bridge
CBA	chronic bronchitis and asthma
CBC	complete blood count;
CBD	common bile duct; closed bladder drainage; cannabidial
CBF	cerebral blood flow
CBFS	cerebral blood flow studies
CBFV	cerebral blood flow velocity
CBG	capillary blood glucose
CBI	continuous bladder irrigation
CBN	chronic benign neutropenia
CBR	complete bedrest; chronic bedrest; carotid bodies resected
CBS	chronic brain syndrome
CC	chief complaint; cubic centimeter; critical condition; creatinine clearance; cerebral concussion; chronic complainer; clean catch (urine); cord compression
CCA	common carotid artery
CCAP	capsule cartilage articular preservation
CC & C	colony count and culture
CCE	clubbing, cyanosis, and edema
CCF	compound comminuted fracture; crystal-induced chemostatic factor

CCHD	cyanotic congenital heart disease
CCI	chronic coronary insufficiency
CCMSU	clean catch midstream urine
CCNS	cell cycle nonspecific
C-collar	cervical collar
CCPD	continuous cycling/cyclical peritoneal dialysis
CCR	continuous complete remission
CCRU	critial care recovery unit
CCS	cell cycle specific; Cooperative Care Suite
CCT	congenitally corrected transposition
CCTGA	congenitally corrected transposition of the great arteries
CCTV	closed circuit television
CCU	coronary care unit
CCUP	colpocystourethropexy
CCX	complications
CD	Crohn's disease; cesarean delivery; continuous drainage
C/D	cup to disc ratio
C & D	cytoscopy and dilatation; curettage and desiccation
CDA	congenital dyserythropoietic anemia
CDAI	Crohn's Disease Activity Index
CDB	cough, deep breathe
CDC	Cancer Detection Center; calculated day of confinement
CDE	common duct exploration
CDH	congenital dysplasia of the hip; chronic daily headache
CDLE	chronic discoid lupus erythematosus
cdyn	dynamic compliance
CE	cardiac enlargement; contrast echocardiology; central episiotomy; continuing education
CEA	carotid endarterectomy; carcinoembryonic antigen
CECT	contrast enhancement computed tomography

CEI	continuous extravascular infusion
CEO	chief executive officer
CEP	congenital erythropoietic porphyria; countercurrent electrophoresis
CEPH	cephalic
CEPH Floc	cephalin flocculation
CE & R	central episiotomy and repair
CERA	cortical evoked response audiometry
CERV	cervical
CES	cognitive environmental stimulation
CF	cystic fibrosis; Caucasian female; complement fixation; cardiac failure; cancer-free; count fingers; Christmas factor; contractile force
CFA	common femoral artery; complete Freund's adjuvant
CFIDS	chronic fatigue and immune dysfunction syndrome
CFM	close fitting mask
CFP	cystic fibrosis protein
CFS	cancer family syndrome
CFT	complement fixation test
CF test	complement fixation test
CFU	colony forming units
CFU-S	colony forming unit - spleen
CG	cholecystogram
CGB	chronic gastrointestinal bleeding
CGD	chronic granulomatous disease
CGI	Clinical Global Impression (scale)
CGL	chronic granulocytic leukemia; with correction/with glasses
CGN	chronic glomerulonephritis
CGTT	cortisol glucose tolerance test
CH	child; chronic; chest; chief; crown-heel; convalescent hospital; cluster headache
CHAI	continuous hepatic artery infusion
CHB	complete heart block
CHD	congenital heart disease; childhood diseases
CHF	congestive heart failure; Crimean hemorrhagic fever
CHFV	combined high frequency of ventilation
CHI	closed head injury
CHO	carbohydrate
chol	cholesterol
chr	chronic
CHRS	congenital hereditary retinoschisis
CHS	Chediak-Higashi syndrome
CHU	closed head unit
CI	cardiac index; cesium implant; complete iridectomy
CI	curie(s)
CIA	chronic idiopathic anhidrosis
CIAED	collagen induced autoimmune ear disease
CIB	cytomegalic inclusion bodies
CIBD	chronic inflammatory bowel disease
CIC	circulating immune complexes
CICE	combined intracapsular cataract extraction
CICU	cardiac intensive care unit
CID	cytomegalic inclusion disease
CIDP	chronic inflammatory dymelinating polyradineuropathy
CIDS	continuous insulin delivery system; cellular immunodeficiency syndrome
CIE	counterimmunoelectrophoresis; crossed immunoelectrophoresis
CIN	chronic interstitial nephritis; cervical intraepithelial neoplasia
CIrc	circumcision; circumference; circulation
CIS	carcinoma in situ
CIU	chronic idiopathic urticaria
CJD	Creutzfeldt-Jakob disease
Ck	check; creatinine kinase
CK-MB	a creatine kinase isoenzyme
cl	cloudy

CL	critical list
CLA	community living arrangements
clav	clavicle
CLBBB	complete left bundle branch block
CLC	cork leather and celastic (orthotic)
CLD	chronic lung disease
CLF	cholesterol-lecithin flocculation
CLH	chronic lobular hepatitis
CLL	chronic lymphocytic leukemia
CLLE	columnar-lined lower esophagus
cl llq	clear liquid
CLO	cod liver oil; close
CL & P	cleft lip and palate
CIH	hepatic clearance
CLT	chronic lymphocytic thyroiditis
CI VOID	clean voided specimen
clysis	hypodermoclysis
cm	centimeter
CM	Caucasian male; costal margin; continuous murmur; contrast media; centimeter; cochlear microphonics; culture media; common migraine
CMBBT	cervical mucous basal body temperature
CMC	chronic mucocutaneous moniliasis
CME	continuing medical education; cystoid macular edema
CMG	cystometrogram
CMHC	Community Mental Health Center
CMHN	Community Mental Health Nurse
CMI	cell-mediated immunity; Cornell Medical Index
CMJ	carpometacarpal joint
CMK	congenital multicystic kidney
CML	cell-mediated lympholysis; chronic myelogenous leukemia
CMM	cutaneous malignant melanoma

CMRNG	chromosomally resistant Neisseria gonorrhoeae
CMRO$_2$	cerebral metabolic rate for oxygen
CMS	circulation motion sensation
CMSUA	clean midstream urinalysis
CMV	cytomegalovirus; cool mist vaporizer; controlled mechanical ventilation
CN	cranial nerve
CNA	chart not available
CNH	central neurogenic hypernea
CNS	central nervous system; clinical nurse specialist
C/O	complains of; complaints; under care of
CO	cardiac output; carbon monoxide
Co	cobalt
CO$_2$	carbon dioxide
CoA	coarctation of the aorta
COAD	chronic obstructive airway disease; chronic obstructive arterial disease
COAG	chronic open angle glaucoma
COC	combination oral contraceptive
COD	cause of death
COEPS	cortically originating extrapyramidal symptoms
COG	cognitive function tests; Central Oncology Group
COH	carbohydrate
Coke	Coca-Cola
Collyr	eye wash
col/ml	colonies per milliliter
COLD	chronic obstructive lung disease
COLD A	cold agglutin titer
COMP	complications; compound
conc	concentrated
CONG	congenital
COPD	chronic obstructive pulmonary disease
COPE	chronic obstructive pulmonary emphysema
cor	coronary
COT	content of thought
COTX	cast off to x-ray

COU	cardiac observation unit
CP	cerebral palsy; cleft palate; creatine phosphokinase; chest pain; chronic pain; chondromalacia patella
C & P	cystoscopy and pyelography
CPA	costophrenic angle; cardiopulmonary arrest; cerebellar pontile angle
CPAF	chlorpropamide-alcohol flush
CPAP	continuous positive airway pressure
CPB	cardiopulmonary bypass
CPBA	competitive protein-binding assay
CPC	clinicopathologic conference; cerebral palsy clinic
CPCR	cardiopulmonary-cerebral resuscitation
CPD	chorioretinopathy and pituitary dysfunction; cephalopelvic disproportion; chronic peritoneal dialysis
CPDD	calcium pyrophosphate deposition disease
CPE	chronic pulmonary emphysema; cardiogenic pulmonary edema
CPGN	chronic progressive glomerulonephritis
CPH	chronic persistent hepatitis
CPI	constitutionally psychopathia inferior
CPID	chronic pelvic inflammatory disease
CPK	creatinine phosphokinase
CPKD	childhood polycystic kidney disease
CPL	criminal procedure law
CPM	central pontine myelinolysis; continuous passive motion; continue present management; counts per minute
CPmax	peak serum concentration
CPmin	trough serum concentration
CPN	chronic pyelonephritis
CPP	cerebral perfusion pressure
CPPB	continuous positive pressure breathing
CPPV	continuous positive pressure ventilation
CPR	cardiopulmonary resuscitation
CPS	complex partial seizures
CPT	chest physiotherapy
CPTH	chronic post-traumatic headache
Cr	creatinine
CR	cardiorespiratory; controlled release; cardiac rehabilitation; colon resection; closed reduction; complete remission
CRA	central retinal artery
CRAO	central retinal artery occlusion
CRBBB	complete right bundle branch block
CRC	colorectal cancer
CrCl	creatinine clearance
CRD	chronic renal disease
CREST	calcinosis, Raynaud's phenomenon, esophageal dysmotility, sclerodactyly and telangiectasia
CRF	chronic renal failure; corticotropin-releasing factor
CRI	chronic renal insufficiency
CRIE	crossed radioimmuno-electrophoresis
crit	hematocrit
CRL	crown rump length
CRO	cathode ray oscilloscope
CRP	C-reactive protein
CRPF	chloroquine-resistant plasmodium falciparum
CRST	calcification, Raynaud's phenomenon, scleroderma and telangiectasia
CRT	copper reduction test; cathode ray tube; central reaction time; cadaver renal transplant
CrTr	crutch training
CRTX	cast removed take x-ray
CRVO	central retinal vein occlusion

CS	coronary sclerosis; central supply; clinical stage; conjunctiva-sclera; consciousness; cat scratch
C & S	culture and sensitivity
C/S	cesarean section; culture and sensitivity
CSBF	coronary sinus blood flow
CSC	cornea, sclera, conjunctiva
CS & CC	culture, sensitivity, and colony count
CSD	cat scratch disease
CSE	cross-section echocardiography
C sect	cesarean section
CSF	cerebrospinal fluid; colony-stimulating factor
C-Sh	chair shower
CSH	carotid sinus hypersensitivity
CSICU	cardiac surgery intensive care unit
CSH	continuous subcutaneous insulin infusion
CS IV	clinical stage 4
CSLU	chronic status leg ulcer
CSM	circulation, sensation, movement; cerebrospinal meningitis
CSOM	chronic serous otitis media
CSP	cellulose sodium phosphate
CSR	Cheyne-Stokes respiration; central supply room; corrective septorhinoplasty
CST	convulsive shock therapy; contraction stress test; cosyntropin stimulation test
CSU	cardiac surveillance unit; cardiovascular surgery unit
CT	computed tomography; circulation time; coagulation time; clotting time; corneal thickness; cervical traction; Coomb's test; cardiothoracic; coated tablet
Cta	catamenia (menses)
CTB	ceased to breathe
CT & DB	cough, turn, and deep breathe
CTD	chest tube drainage

CTF	Colorado tick fever
CTL	cytotoxic T lymphocytes
CT/MPR	computed tomography with multiplanar reconstructions
cTNM	clinical-diagnostic staging of cancer
CTP	comprehensive treatment plan
CTR	carpal tunnel release
CTS	carpal tunnel syndrome
CTSP	called to see patient
CTW	central terminal of Wilson
CTXN	contraception
CTZ	chemoreceptor trigger zone
Cu	copper
CU	cause unknown
CUC	chronic ulcerative colitis
CUD	cause undetermined
CUG	cystourethrogram
CUS	chronic undifferentiated schizophrenia
CUSA	Cavitron® ultrasonic aspirator
CV	cardiovascular; cell volume
CVA	cerebrovsascular accident; costovertebral angle
CVAT	costovertebral angle tenderness
CVC	central venous catheter
CVD	collagen vascular disease
CVI	cerebrovascular insufficiency; continuous venous infusion
CVID	common variable immune deficiency
CVO	central vein occlusion; conjugate diamater of pelvic inlet
CVP	central venous pressure
CVRI	coronary vascular resistance index
CVS	clean voided specimen; cardiovascular system; chorionic villus sampling
CVUG	cysto-void urethrogram
C/W	consistent with; crutch walking
CWE	cottonwool exudates
CWMS	color, warmth, movement sensation
CWP	coal worker's pneumoconiosis
CWS	cotton wool spots

Cx	cervix; culture; cancel	**DDS**	dialysis disequilibrium syndrome;
CxMT	cervical motion tenderness		
CXR	chest x-ray	**DDST**	Denver Development Screening Test
CYSTO	cystoscopy; cystogram		
		DDx	differential diagnosis
D	diarrhea; day; divorced; distal; dead; right; diopter	**D & E**	dilation and evacuation
		DEC	decrease
D1,D2	dorsal vertebra #1, #2	**decub**	decubitus
DA	direct admission	**DEF**	decayed, extracted or filled
DAD	drug administration device	**degen**	degenerative
DAI	diffuse axonal injury	**del**	delivery, delivered
DAH	disordered action of the heart	**DEP ST SEG**	depressed ST segment
DAL	drug analysis laboratory	**DER**	disulfiram-ethanol reaction
DANA	drug induced antinuclear antibodies	**DES**	disequilibrium syndrome; diffuse esophageal spasm
DAT	direct agglutination test; diet as tolerated; dementia of the Alzheimer type	**DEV**	duck embryo vaccine; deviation
		DEVR	dominant exudative vitreoretinopathy
DAW	dispense as written		
DAWN	Drug Abuse Warning Network	**dex.**	dexter (right)
dB	decibel	**DF**	decayed and filled
DB	date of birth	**DFD**	defined formula diets
DB & C	deep breathing and coughing	**DFE**	distal femoral epiphysis
DBE	deep breathing exercise	**DFMC**	daily fetal movement count
DBIL	direct bilirubin	**DFR**	diabetic floor routine
DBP	diastolic blood pressure	**DFU**	dead fetus in uterus
DBS	diminished breath sounds	**DGI**	disseminated gonococcal infection
D & C	dilation and curettage		
DC,d/c	discontinue; discharge; decrease; diagonal conjugate	**DGM**	ductal glandular mastectomy
		DH	developmental history; diaphragmatic hernia; delayed hypersensitivity
DCH	delayed cutaneous hypersensitivity		
DCO	diffusing capacity of carbon monoxide	**DHBV**	duck hepatitis B virus
		DHF	dengue hemorrhagic fever
DCR	delayed cutaneous reaction	**DHL**	diffuse histocytic lymphoma
DCSA	double contrast shoulder arthrography	**DHS**	duration of hospital stay
		DI	diabetes insipidus; detruosor instability
DCT	direct (antiglobulin) Coombs test; deep chest therapy		
		dlag	diagnosis
DCTM	delay computer tomographic myelography	**Dlath SW**	diathermy short wave
		DIC	Drug Information Center; disseminated intravascular coagulation
DD	differential diagnosis; down drain; dependent drainage; dry dressing; Duchenne's dystrophy		
		DIE	die in emergency department
		DIFF	differential blood ocunt
D & D	diarrhea and dehydration	**DIJOA**	dominantly inherited juvenile optic atrophy
DDD	degenerative disc disease; dense deposit (renal)disease		
		dil	dilute

DILD	diffuse infiltrative lung disease	DNR	do not resuscitate/ report
DILE	drug induced lupus erythematosus	DNS	do not show; deviated nasal septum; dysplastic nevus syndrome
dim	diminish		
DIMOAD	diabetes insipidus, diabetes mellitus, optic atrophy and deafness	DO	right eye
		DOA	dead on arrival; date of admission
DIP	distal interphalangeal; desquamative interstitial pneumonia; drip infusion pyelogram	DOA-DRA	dead on arrival; despite resuscitative attempts
		DOB	date of birth; doctor's order book
dis	dislocation	DOC	drug of choice; died of other causes
DIS	Diagnostic Interview Schedule questionnaire		
		DOE	dyspnea on exertion
disch	discharge	DOI	date of injury
DISH	diffuse idiopathic skeletal hyperostosis	DOLV	double outlet left ventricle
		DORV	double-outlet right ventricle
dist	distilled	DORx	date of treatment
DIV	double inlet ventricle	DOT	Doppler ophthalmic test; died on table
DIVA	digital intravenous angiography	DP	dorsalis pedis (pulse); diastolic pressure
DJD	degenerative joint disease		
DK	diabetic ketoacidosis; dark	DPC	discharge planning coordinator; delayed primary closure
DKA	diabetic ketoacidosis		
dl	deciliter		
DL	danger list; deciliter; direct laryngoscopy; diagnostic laparoscopy	DPDL	diffuse poorly differentiated lymphocytic lymphoma
		DPM	disintegrations per minute
DLE	discoid lupus erythematosus	DPV	delayed pressure urticaria
DLIS	digitalis-like immunoreactive substance	DR	delivery room; diabetic retinopathy
DLMP	date of last menstrual period	DREZ	dorsal root entry zone
DLNMP	date of last normal menstrual period	DRG	diagnosis-related groups
		DRSG	dressing
DM	diabetes mellitus; diastolic murmur; dermatomyositis	DS	discharge summary; Down's syndrome; double strength; disoriented; dextrose stick
DMD	Duchenne's muscular dystrophy		
		DSA	digital subtraction angiography
DME	durable medical equipment	DSD	dry sterile dressing; discharge summary dictated
DMF	decayed, missing or filled		
DMKA	diabetes mellitus ketoacidosis	dsg	dressing
DMOOC	diabetes mellitus out of control	DSI	deep shock insulin
DMX	diathermy, massage and exercise	DSM	drink skim milk; Diagnostic & Statistical Manual
DN	down	DSS	dengue shock syndrome
DNI	do not intubate	DST	dexamethasone suppression test; donor specific transfusion
DNKA	did not keep appointment		
DNP	do not publish		

DT	delirium tremens; discharge tomorrow	ECBD	exploration of common bile duct
DTD #30	dispense 30 such doses	ECC	emergency cardiac care; endocervical curettage
DTH	delayed-type hypersensitivity		
DTR	deep tendon reflexes	ECCE	extracapsular cataract extraction
DTs	delerium tremens		
DTS	donor specific transfusion	ECD	endocardial cushion defect
DTT	diphtheria tetanus toxoid	ECEMG	evoked compound electromyography
DTV	due to void		
DTX	detoxification	ECF	extracellular fluid; extended care facility; eosinophilic chemostactic factor
DU	duodenal ulcer; duroxide uptake; diabetic urine; diagnosis undetermined		
		ECG	electrocardiogram
DUB	dysfunctional uterine bleeding	ECHO	echocardiogram
DUE	drug use evaluation	ECL	extent of cerebral lesion; extracapillary lesions
DUI	driving under the influence		
DUR	drug utilization review	ECM	erythema chronicum migrans
DVD	dissociated vertical deviation	ECMO	extracorporeal membrane oxygenation
DVIU	direct vision internal urethrotomy		
		ECN	extended care nursery
DVR	double valve replacement	ECR	emergency chemical restraint
DVT	deep vein thrombosis	ECRL	extensor carpi radialis longus
DW	dextrose in water; distilled water; deionized water	ECT	electroconvulsive therapy; enhanced computer tomography; emission computed tomography
DWDL	diffuse well differentiated lymphocytic lymphoma		
Dx	diagnosis		
Dz	disease; dozen	ECU	extensor carpi ulnaris
		ECW	extracellular water
E	edema	ED	emergency department; epidural
4E	4 plus edema		
E>A	say EEE, comes out as A,A,A upon auscultation of lung, showing consolidation	ED50	median effective dose
		EDC	estimated date of confinement; estimated date of conception; end diastolic counts; digitorium communis
EAA	electrothermal atomic absorption		
EAC	external auditory canal	EDD	expected date of delivery
EAHF	eczema, allergy, hay fever	EDM	early diastolic murmur
EAM	external auditory meatus	EDS	Ehler-Danlos syndrome
EAST	external rotation, abduction stress test	EDV	end-diastolic volume
		EE	equine encephalitis; end to end
EAT	ectopic atrial tachycardia		
EB	epidermolysis bullosa	EEE	Eastern equine encephalomyelitis; edema, erythema and exudate
EBL	estimated blood loss		
EBV	Epstein-Barr virus		
EC	enteric coated; eyes closed; extracellular	EEG	electroencephalogram
		EENT	eyes, ears, nose, throat

EF	extended-field (radiotherapy); endurance factor; ejection fraction
EFAD	essential fatty acid deficiency
EFE	endocardial fibroelastosis
EFM	external fetal monitoring
EFW	estimated fetal weight
EGA	estimated gestational age
EGBUS	external genitalia, Bartholin, urethral, Skene's glands
EGD	esophagogastroduodenoscopy
EGF	epidermal growth factor
EGTA	esophageal gastric tube airway
EH	essential hypertension; enlarged heart; extramedullary hematopoiesis
EHB	elevate head of bed
EHF	epidemic hemorrhagic fever
E & I	endocrine and infertility
EIA	exercise induced asthma
EIAB	extracranial-intracranial arterial bypass
EIB	exercise induced bronchospasm
EID	electronic infusion device
EIF	eukaryotic initiation factor
EIS	endoscopic injection scleropathy
EJ	external jugular; elbow jerk
EKC	epidemic keratoconjunctivitis
EKG	electrocardiogram
EKY	electrokymogram
E-L	external lids
ELF	elective low forceps
ELH	endolymphatic hydrops
ELISA	enzyme-linked immunosorbent assay
elix	elixir
ELOP	estimated length of program
ELP	electrophoresis
EM	electron microscope; ejection murmur; erythema multiforme
EMB	endomyocardial biopsy
EMC	encephalomyocarditis
EMD	electromechanical dissociation

EMF	erythrocyte maturation factor; evaporated milk formula
EMG	electromyography; essential monoclonal gammopathy
EMIC	emergency maternity and infant care
E-MICR	electron microscopy
EMIT	enzyme multiplied immunoassay technique
EMR	emergency mechanical restraint; empty, measure and record; educable mentally retarded
EMS	emergency medical services
EMT	emergency medical technician
EMV	eye, motor, verbal
EMW	electromagnetic waves
ENA	extractable nuclear antigen
ENDO	endotracheal
ENG	electronystagmography
ENL	erythema nodosum leprosum
ENP	extractable nucleoprotein
ENT	ears, nose, throat
EO	eyes open
EOA	examine, opinion, and advice; esophageal obturator airway
EOG	electro-oculogram; Ethrane®, oxygen and gas
EOM	extraocular movement; extraocular muscles
EOMI	extraocular muscles intact
EORA	elderly onset rheumatoid arthritis
eos	eosinophil
EP	endogenous pyrogen; electrophysiologic
EPA	eicosapentaenoic acid
EPB	extensor pollicis brevis
EPIS	episiotomy
eplth	epithelial
EPL	extensor pollicis longus
EPM	electronic pacemaker
EPO	recombinant human erythropoietin
EPP	erythropoietic protoporphyria
EPR	electrophrenic respiration; emergency physical restraint

EPS	electrophysiologic study; extrapyramidal syndrome/symptoms
EPT®	early pregnancy test
EPTS	existed prior to service
ER	emergency room; estrogen receptor; external rotation
ERA	evoked response audiometry; estrogen receptor assay
ERCP	endoscopic retrograde cholangiopancreatography
ERFC	erythrocyte rosette forming cells
ERG	electroretinogram
ERL	effective refractory length
ERP	estrogen receptor protein; endoscopic retrograde pancreatography
ERPF	effective renal plasma flow
ERT	estrogen replacement therapy
ERV	expiratory reserve volume
ESAP	evoked sensory (nerve) action potentiation
ESC	end systolic counts
ESM	ejection systolic murmur
ESP	end systolic pressure
ESR	erythrocyte sedimentation rate
ESRD	end-stage renal disease
ess	essential
EST	electroshock therapy
ESWL	extracorporeal shockwave lithotripsy
ET	endotracheal; esotropia; eustachian tube; ejection time; exercise treadmill
et	and
et al	and others
ETF	eustachian tubal function
EtO	estimated time of ovulation
ETT	endotracheal tube; exercise tolerance test
EU	excretory urography
EUA	examine under anesthesia
EVAC	evacuation
eval	evaluate
EWB	estrogen withdrawal bleeding
EWSCLs	extended-wear soft contact lenses

exam	examination
EXP	exploration; experienced
exp lap	exploratory laparotomy
ext	extract; external
ext rot	external rotation
EX U	excretory urogram
F	Fahrenheit; female; flow; facial; firm; French
F1	offspring from first generation
F2	offspring from second generation
FA	folic acid; femoral artery
FAAP	family assessment adjustment pass
FAC	fractional area concentration
FACH	forceps to after-coming head
FAD	Family Assessment Device
FAI	functional assessment inventory
FALL	fallopian
FAM	family
FANA	fluorescent antinuclear antibody
FAP	fibrillating action potential; familial amyloid polyneuropathy
FAS	fetal alcohol syndrome
FAST	functional assessment staging (of Alzheimer's disease); fluoro-allergo sorbent test
FAT	fluorescent antibody test
FB	fasting blood sugar; foreign body; finger breadth
FBS	fasting blood sugar; fetal bovine serum
FBU	fingers below umbilicus
FBW	fasting blood work
FC	foley catheter; finger counting
FC	foley catheter; fever, chills
F+C	flare and cells
F & C	foam and condom
F cath	foley catheter
FCC	follicular center cells; familial colonic cancer; fracture compound comminuted
FCDB	fibrocystic disease of the breast

FCH	familial combined hyperlipidemia	**FHT**	fetal heart tone
FCMC	family centered maternity care	**FiCO$_2$**	fraction of inspired carbon dioxide
FCMD	Fukiyama's congenital muscular dystrophy	**FiO$_2$**	fraction of inspired oxygen
		FL	fluid
FCMN	family centered maternity nursing	**FLK**	funny looking kid
		FLS	flashing lights and/or scotoma
FCR	flexor carpi radialis	**FM**	fetal movements; face mask
FCRB	flexor carpi radialis brevis	**F & M**	firm and midline (uterus)
FCSNVD	fever, chills, sweating, nausea, vomiting, diarrhea	**FMC**	fetal movement count
		FMD	ffoot and mouth disease
FCU	flexor carpi ulnaris	**FME**	full mouth extraction
FD	focal distrance; familial dysautonomia	**FMF**	forced midexpiratory flow; familial Mediterranean fever
F & D	fixed and dilated	**FMG**	foreign medical graduate; fine mesh gauze
FDA	fronto-dextra anterior		
FDIU	fetal death in utero	**FMH**	family medical history; fibromuscular hyperplasia
FDP	fibrin-degradation products; flexor digitorum profundus	**FMP**	fasting metabolic panel
FDS	flexor digitorum superficialis; for duration of stay	**FMX**	full mouth x-ray
		FN	false negative; finger-to-nose
Fe	iron; female	**FNAB**	fine-needle aspiration biopsy
FEC	forced expiratory capacity	**FNAC**	fine-needle aspiration cytology
FEF	forced expiratory flow	**FNCJ**	fine needle catheter jejunostomy
FEL	familial erythrophagocytic lymphohistiocytosis		
		FNH	focal nodular hyperplasia
FEM	femoral	**FNR**	false negative rate
Fem-pop	femoral popliteal (bypass)	**FNS**	functional neuromuscular stimulation
FEN	fluid, electrolytes, nutrition		
FENa	fractional extraction of sodium	**FOB**	foot of bed; fiberoptic bronchoscope; father of baby
FEP	free erythrocyte protoporphorin		
FEV	forced expiratory volume	**FOBT**	fecal occult blood test
FF	filtration fraction; fundus firm; flat feet; fat free; force fluids	**FOC**	father of child
		FOD	free of disease
FFA	free fatty acid	**FOI**	flight of ideas
F factor	fertility/sex factor	**FOOB**	fell out of bed
FFP	fresh frozen plasma	**FP**	family planning; family practice; frozen plasma; flat plate; false positive
FGF	fibroblast growth factor		
FH	family history; fetal heart; fundal height		
		FPAL	fullterm, premature, abortion, living
FHF	fulminant hepatic failure		
FHH	familial hypocalciuric hypercalcemia	**FPB**	flexor pollicis brevis
		FPD	feto-pelvic disporportion; fixed partial denture
FHI	Fuch's heterochromic iridocyclitis		
		FPG	fasting plasma glucose
FHR	fetal heart rate	**FPIA**	fluorescence-polarization immunoassay
FHS	fetal heart sounds; fetal hydantoin syndrome		
		FPL	flexor pollicis longus

FPL	flexor pollicis longus		**Fx**	fracture; fractional urine
FPNA	first-pass nuclear angiocardiography		**Fx-dis**	fracture-dislocation
			FXN	function
FR	flow rate		**FXR**	fracture
F & R	flow and rhythm (pulse)			
FRC	functional residual capacity		**G**	gauge; gravida; gram; gallop
FRJM	full range of joint motion		**G1-4**	grade 1-4
RROM	full range of movement		**GA**	gastric analysis; general appearance; general anesthesia; gestational age
FS	frozen section; flexible sigmoidoscopy			
FSB	fetal scalp blood		**GABA**	gamma-aminobutyric acid
FSBM	full strength breast milk		**GABHS**	group A beta hemolytic streptococci
FSE	fetal scalp electrode			
FSG	focal and segmental		**GAD**	generalized anxiety disorder
FSGS	focal and segmental glomerulosclerosis		**GAS**	general adaption syndrome
			GAT	group adjustment therapy
FSH	follicle stimulating hormone; facioscapulohumeral		**GB**	gallbladder
			GBM	glomerular basement membrane
FSHMD	facioscapulohumeral muscular dystrophy			
			GBP	gastric bypass
FSHRF	follicle stimulating hormone releasing factor		**GBS**	gallbladder series; Guillain-Barre syndrome; group B streptococci
FSP	fibrin split products			
FT	full term		**GC**	gonococci (gonorrhea); geriatric chair
FTA	fluorescent treponemal/titer antibody			
			G-C	gram-negative cocci
FTD	failure to descend		**G+C**	gram-positive cocci
FTI	free thyroxine index		**GCDFP**	gross cystic disease fluid protein
FTLFC	full term living female child			
FTLMC	full term living male child		**GCIIS**	glucose control insulin infusion system
FTN	finger-to-nose; full term nursery			
			GCS	Glasgow coma scale
FTND	full-term normal delivery		**GCT**	giant cell tumor
FTP	failure to progress		**GD**	Graves disease
FTR	for the record		**G & D**	growth and development
FTSG	full-thickness skin graft		**GDF**	gel diffusion precipitin
FTT	failure to thrive		**GDM**	gestational diabetes mellitus
F & U	flanks and upper quadrants		**GE**	gastroenteritis
F/U	follow-up; fundus at umbilicus		**GEP**	gastroenteropancreatic
FUB	functional uterine bleeding		**GER**	gastroesophageal reflux
FUN	follow-up note		**GERD**	gastroesophageal reflux disease
FUO	fever of undetermined origin			
FVC	forced vital capacity		**GETA**	general endotracheal anesthesia
FVH	focal vascular headache			
FVL	flow volume loop		**GF**	grandfather; gluten-free; gastric fistula
FWB	full weight bearing			
FWS	fetal warfarin syndrome		**GFR**	glomerular filtration rate
FWW	front wheel walker		**GG**	gamma globulin

GGE	generalized glandular enlargement
GGT	gamma glutamyl transpeptidase
GGTP	gamma glutamyl transpeptidase
GH	growth hormone
GHb	glycosylated hemoglobin
GHD	growth hormone deficiency
GHQ	general health questionnaire
GI	gastrointestinal; granuloma inguinale
GIB	gastric ileal bypass
GIC	general immunocompetence
GIFT	gamete intrafallopian treatment
GIP	giant cell interstitial pneumonia; gastric inhibitory peptide
GIS	gastrointestinal series
GIT	gastrointestinal tract
GJ	gastrojejunostomy
GL	greatest length
GLA	gingivolinguoaxial
GLNH	giant lymph node hyperplasia
GM	gram; grandmother
GMC	general medicine clinic
GMTs	geometric mean antibody titers
GN	glomerulonephritis; gram negative; graduate nurse
GnRH	gonadotropin-releasing hormone
GOT	glucose oxidase test
GP	general practitioner; gutta percha
G/P	gravida/para
GPC	gram positive cocci; giant papillary conjunctivitis
G6PD	glucose-6-phosphate dehydrogenase
GPMAL	gravida, para, multiple births, abortions and live births
GPN	graduate practical nurse
gr	grain
G-R	gram-negative rods
G+R	gram-positive rods
grav	gravid (pregnant)
GRD	gastroesophageal reflux disease

GRN	granules
GSC	Glasgow coma scale
GSD	glucogen storage disease
GSD-1	glycogen storage disease, type 1
GSE	grip strong and equal; gluten sensitive enteropathy
GSI	genuine stress incontinence
GSP	general survey panel
GSPN	greater superficial petrosal neurectomy
GSR	galvanic skin resistance
GSW	gunshot wound
GT	gastrotomy tube; gait training
GTN	gestational trophoblastic neoplasms
GTT	glucose tolerance test; drop
GU	genitourinary
GUS	genitourinary sphincter; genitourinary system
GVF	good visual fields
GVHD	graft-versus-host disease
G & W	glycerin and water
GW	glucose in water
GWA	gunshot wound of the abdomen
GWT	gunshot wound of the throat
GXT	graded exercise testing
GYN	gynecology
H	hypodermic; hydrogen; hour; husband
H_2	histamine
HA	headache; hyperalimentation; hypothalmic amenorrhea; hearing aid; hemolytic anemia; hospital admission; hepatitis, type A
HAA	hepatitis-associated antigen
HAE	hereditary angioedema; hepatic artery embolization; hearing aid evaluation
HAI	hepatic arterial infusion
HAL	hyperalimentation
HAN	heroin associated nephropathy
HANE	hereditary angioneurotic edema

HAPS	hepatic arterial perfusion scintigraphy
HAQ	Headache Assessment Questionnaire
HAS	hyperalimentation solution
HASHD	hypertensive arteriosclerotic heart disease
HAT	head, arms, and trunk
HAV	hepatitis A virus; hallux abducto valgus
HB	hemoglobin; heart block; hepatitis, type B; hold breakfast
HBBW	hold breakfast blood work
HBD	has been drinking
HBGM	home blood glucose monitoring
HBI	hemibody irradiation
HBIG	hepatitis B immune globulin
HbAlc	glycosylated hemoglobin
HBF	hepatic blood flow
HBO	hyperbaric oxygen
HBP	high blood pressure
HBS	Health Behavior Scale
HBsAg	hepatitis B surface antigen
HBV	hepatitis B virus; hepatitis B vaccine; honeybee venom
HC	home care; head circumference; heel cord; house call; Hickman catheter
HCA	health care aide
HCC	hepatocellular carcinoma
HCL	hair cell leukemia
HCLs	hard contact lenses
HCM	health care maintenance; hypertropic cardiomyopathy
HCP	hereditoary coporphyria
HCT	hematocrit; histamine challenge test
HCVD	hypertensive cardiovascular disease
HD	Hodgkin's disease; Huntington's disease; hearing distance; hemodialysis; helloma mole; hip disarticulation; high dose
HDCV	human diploid cell vaccine
HDL	high-density lipoprotein
HDLW	hearing distance for watch in left ear
HDRW	hearing distance for watch in right ear
HDN	hemolytic disease of the newborn
HDPAA	heparin-dependent platelet-associated antibody
HDRS	Hamilton Depression Rate Scale
H & E	hemorrhage and exudate; hematoxylin and eosin
HEENT	head, eyes, ears, nose and throat
HEK	human embryonic kidney
HEL	human embryonic lung
hemi	hemiplegia
HEMPAS	hereditary erythrocytic multinuclearity with positive acidified serum test
HEP	histamine equivalent prick; hepatic
HES	hypereosinophilic syndrome
HF	heart failure
HFD	high forceps delivery
HFHL	high frequency hearing loss
Hbg	hemoglobin
HGH	human growth hormone
HH	hiatal hernia; hypogonadotrophic hypogonadism; home health; hard of hearing
H & H	hematocrit and hemoglobin
HHC	home health care
HHD	hypertensive heart disease
HHFM	high humidity face mask
HHN	hand held nebulizer
HHNK	hyperglycemic hyperosmolar nonketotic (coma)
HHT	hereditary hemorrhagic telangiectasis
HHV-6	human herpes virus 6
HI	hemagglutination inhibition; head injury
HIA	hemagglutination inhibition antibody
HIB	Haemophilus influenzae type B (vaccine)

HID	headache, insomnia, depression
HIE	hypoxic-ischemic encephalopathy
HIF	higher integrative functions
HIL	hypoxic-ischemic lesion
HIR	head injury routine
HIS	Health Intention Scale
Histo	histoplasmin skin test
HIT	heparin induced thrombocytopenia; histamine inhalation test
HIV	human immunodeficiency virus
HIVD	herniated intervertebral disc
HJR	hepato-jugular reflex
H-K	hand to knee
HKAFO	hip-knee-ankle-foot orthosis
HKO	hip-knee orthosis
HL	heparin lock; harelip; hairline; hearing level; Hickman line;
HLA	human lymphocyte antigen
HLD	herniated lumbar disc
HLHS	hypoplastic left heart syndrome
HLV	hypoplatic left ventricle
HM	hand motion
HMD	hyaline membrane disease
HMG	human menopausal gonadotropin
HMI	healed myocardial infarction
HMP	hot moist packs
HMR	histocytic medullary reticulosis
HMX	heat massage exercise
HN	high nitrogen
H & N	head and neck
HNP	herniated nucleus pulposis
HNRNA	heterogeneous nuclear ribonucleic acid
HNV	has not voided
HO	house officer
H/O	history of
H_2O	water
HOB	head of bed
HOB UPSOB	head of bed up for shortness of breath
HOC	Health Officer Certificate
HOCM	hypertrophic obstructive cardiomyopathy

HOG	halothane, oxygen and gas (nitrous oxide)
HOH	hard of hearing
HOPI	history of present illness
HP	hemiplegia; hemipelvectomy; hot packs
H & P	history and physical
HPA	human papilloma virus; hypothalamic-pituitary-adrenal (axis)
HPF	high-power field
HPFH	hereditary persistence of fetal hemoglobin
HPI	history of present illness
HPL	human placenta lactogen
HPLC	high-pressure (performance) liquid chromatography
HPG	human pituitary gonadotropin
HPL	hyperplexia; human placental lactogen
HPM	hemiplegic migraine
HPN	home parenteral nutrition
HPO	hypertrophic pulmonary osteoarthropathy; hydrophilic ointment
HPT	hyperparathyroidism
HPZ	high pressure zone
HR	heart rate; hour ; hallux rigidus; hospital record; Harrington rod
HRA	histamine releasing activity
HRLA	human reovirus-like agent
HRS	hepatorenal syndrome
HS	bedtime; hereditary spherocytosis; heel spur; heel stick; herpes simplex; Hartman's (lactated Ringer's) solution
H>S	heel to shin
HSA	human serum albumin; hypersomnia-sleep apnea;
HSBG	heel stick blood gas
HSE	herpes simplex encephalitis
HSG	histosalpingogram
HSM	hepato-splenomegaly; holosystolic murmur
HSP	Henoch-Schonlein purpura
HSR	heated serum reagin

254

HSSE	high soap suds enema
HSV	herpes simplex virus
HT	hypertension; hypermetropia; height; heart; hammertoe; hyperopia; hubbard tank
ht aer	heated aerosol
HTAT	human tetanus antitoxin
HTC	hypertensive crisis
HTF	house tube feeding
HTL	human thymic leukemia
HTLV III	human T cell lymphotrophic virus type III
HTN	hypertension
HTP	House-Tree-Person test
HTVD	hypertensive vascular disease
HUIFM	human leukocyte interferon meloy
HUS	hemolytic uremic syndrome
HV	hallux valgus; has voided
H & V	hemigastrecotomy and vagotomy
HW	heparin well; housewife
hwb	hot water bottle
Hx	history; hospitalization
Hz	Hertz
HZ	herpes zoster
HZO	herpes zoster ophthalmicus
I	independent; impression; incisal; one
IA	intra-amniotic
IAA	interrupted aortic arch
IABC	intra-aortic balloon counterpulsation
IABP	intra-aortic balloon pump
IAC	internal auditory canal
IAC-CPR	interposed abdominal compressions-cardiopulmonary resuscitation
IACP	intra-aortic counterpulsation
IADH	inappropriate antidiuretic hormone
IA DSA	intra-arterial subtraction arteriography
IAHA	immune adherence hemagglutination
IAI	intra-abdominal infection
IAM	internal auditory meatus

IAN	intern admission note
IAP	intermittent acute porphyria
IASD	interatrial septal defect
IAT	indirect antiglobulin test
IB	isolation bed
IBC	iron binding capacity
IBD	inflammatory bowel disease
IBI	intermittent bladder irrigation
ibid	at the same place
IBNR	incurred but not reported
IBS	irritable bowel syndrome
IBW	ideal body weight
IC	irritable colon; intercostal; intracranial; individual counseling
ICA	internal carotid artery; islet cell antibodies
ICBT	intercostobronchial trunk
ICCE	intracapsular cataract extraction
ICCU	intermediate coronary care unit
ICD	instantaneous cardiac death
ICD 9 CM	International Classification of Diseases, 9th Revision, Clinical Modification
ICF	intracellular fluid; intermediate care facility
ICG	indocyanine green
ICH	intracranial hemorrhage
ICM	intracostal margin
ICN	intensive care nursery
ICP	intracranial pressure
ICPP	intubated continuous positive pressure
ICS	intracostal space
ICSH	interstitial cell-stimulating hormone
ICT	intensive conventional therapy; inflammation of connective tissue
ICU	intensive care unit
ICVH	ischemic cerebrovascular headache
ICW	intercellular water
ID	intradermal; initial dose; infectious disease; identification; immunodiffusion; identify

255

I & D	incision and drainage
IDE	Investigational Device Exemption
IDDM	insulin-dependent diabetes mellitus
IDDS	implantable drug delivery system
IDFC	immature dead female child
IDM	infant of a diabetic mother
IDMC	immature dead male child
IDS	Infectious Disease Service
IDV	intermittent demand ventilation
IEC	inpatient exercise center
IEF	iso-electric focusing
IEM	immune electron microscopy
IEP	individualized education program; immunoelectrophoresis
IF	intrinsic factor; immunofluorescence; involved field
IFA	indirect fluorescent antibody test
IgA	immunoglobulin A
IgD	immunoglobulin D
IgE	immunoglobulin E
IGF	insulin-like growth factor
IgG	immunoglobulin G; immune gammaglobulin
IGIV	immune globulin intravenous
IgM	immunoglobulin M
IGR	intrauterine growth retardation
IGT	impaired glucose tolerance
IH	infectious hepatitis; inguinal hernia; indirect hemagglutination
IHA	indirect hemagglutination
IHC	immobilization hypercalcemia
IHD	ischemic heart disease; intrahepatic duct
IHH	idiopathic hypogonadotrophic hypogonadism
IHS	Idiopathic Headache Score
IHs	iris homartomas
IHSS	idiopathic hypertrophic subaortic stenosis
IHT	insulin hypoglycemia test
IICP	increased intracranial pressure
IICU	infant intensive care unit
IJ	internal jugular; ileojejunal
ILD	ischemic leg disease
ILFC	immature living female child
ILM	internal limiting membrane
ILMC	immature living male child
ILMI	inferolateral myocardial infarct
IM	intramuscular; infectious mononucleosis; intermetatarsal; internal medicine
IMA	inferior mesenteric artery; internal mammary artery
IMAG	internal mammary artery graft
IMB	intermenstrual bleeding
IMF	intermaxillary fixation
IMG	internal medicine group (practice)
IMH	indirect microhemagglutination (test)
IMI	inferior myocardial infarction; imipramine
IMIG	intramuscular immunoglobulin
IMN	internal mammary (lymph) node
IMP	impression; impacted
IMV	intermittent mandatory ventilation
IN	interstitial nephritis
INC	incomplete; incontinent; inside-the-needle catheter
IND	investigational new drug
INDM	infant of nondiabetic mother
INF	inferior; infusion; infant; infected
ING	inguinal
Inj	injection; injury
INS	insurance
INST	instrumental delivery
Int	internal
Int-rot	internal rotation
Inver	inversion
I & O	intake and output
IO	intraocular pressure; inferior oblique; initial opening
IOC	intern on call; intraoperative cholangiogram
IOD	interorbital distance

IOF	intraocular fluid	ISH	isolated systolic hypertension
IOFB	intraocular foreign body	ISMA	infantile spinal muscular atrophy
IOH	idiopathic orthostatic hypotension	ISS	Injury Severity Score
IOL	intraocular lens	IST	insulin sensitivity test; insulin shock therapy
ION	ischemic optic neuropathy		
IOP	intraocular pressure	ISW	interstitial water
IORT	intraoperative radiation therapy	IT	intrathecal; inhalation therapy; intertuberous
IOS	intraoperative sonography		
IOV	initial office visit	ITCP	idiopathic thrombocytopenia pupura
IP	intraperitoneal		
IPA	invasive pulmonary aspergillosis	ITE	insufficient therapeutic effect
		ITP	idiopathic thrombocytopenic purpura; interim treatment plan
IPCD	infantile polycystic disease		
IPD	immediate pigment darkening; intermittent peritoneal dialysis		
		ITVAD	indwelling transcutaneous vascular access device
IPFD	intrapartum fetal distress	IU	international unit
IPG	impedance plethysmography; individually polymerized grass	IUCD	intrauterine contraceptive device
		IUD	intrauterine device; intrauterine death
IPJ	interphalangeal joint		
IPK	intractable plantar keratosis	IUFD	intrauterine fetal death
IPMI	inferoposterior myocardial infarct	IUGR	interuterine growth retardation
		IUP	intrauterine pregnancy
IPN	infantile periarteritis nodosa; intern's progress note	IUPD	intrauterine pregnancy delivered
IPP	inflatable penile prosthesis	IV	intravenous
IPPA	inspection, palpation, percussion and auscultation	IVC	intravenous cholangiogram; inferior vena cava; intraventricular catheter
IPPB	intermittent positive pressure breathing		
		IVD	intervertebral disk; intravenous drip
IPPV	intermittent positive pressure ventilation		
		IVDA	intravenous drug abuse
IPV	inactivated polio vaccine	IVF	in vitro fertilization; intravenous fluid
IQ	intelligence quotient		
IR	internal rotation; infrared	IVFE	intravenous fat emulsion
IRBBB	incomplete right bundle branch block	IVGTT	intravenous glucose tolerance test
IRMA	intraretinal microvascular abnormalities	IVH	intravenous hyperalimentation; intraventricular hemorrhage
IRR	intrarenal reflux	IVIG	intravenous immunoglobulin
IRV	inspiratory reserve volume	IVLBW	infant of very low birth weight
IS	intercostal space; incentive spirometer; induced sputum	IVP	intravenous pyelogram; intravenous push
ISB	incentive spirometry breathing	IVPB	intravenous piggyback
ISCs	irreversible sickle cells	IVR	idioventricular rhythm
ISG	immune serum globulin	IVS	intraventricular septum

IVSD	intraventricular septal defect
IVSP	intravenous syringe pump
IVT	intravenous transfusion
IVU	intravenous urography
IWL	insensible water loss
IWMI	inferior wall myocardial infarct
J	joint
JAMG	juvenile autoimmune myasthenia gravis
JC	junior clinicians
JDMS	juvenile dermatomyositis
JE	Japanese encephalitis
JF	joint fluid
JI	jejunoileal
JIB	jejunoileal bypass
JJ	jaw jerk
JMS	junior medical student
JODM	juvenile onset diabetes mellitus
JP	Jobst pump; Jackson-Pratt (drain)
JRA	juvenile rheumatoid arthritis
JSPN	junior student progress note
jt	joint
juv	juvenile
JVD	jugular venous distention
JVP	jugular venous pulse; jugular venous pressure
JVPT	jugular venous pulse tracing
KA	ketoacidosis
KAFO	knee-ankle-foot orthosis
KAO	knee-ankle orthosis
KAS	Katz Adjustment Scale
K Cal	kilocalorie
KCS	keratoconjunctivitis sicca
KD	Kawasaki's disease; knee disarticulation; Keto Diastex®
KDA	known drug allergies
KDDM	kidney disease of diabetes mellitus
KF	kidney function
KFD	Kyasanur Forrest disease
kg	kilogram
K24H	potassium, urine 24 hour
KI	karyopyknotic index
KID	keratitis, ichthyosis, deafness

KILO	kilogram
KISS	saturated solution of potassium iodide
KJ	knee jerk
KK	knee kick
KLH	keyhole limpet hemocyanin (antibody)
KNO	keep needle open
KO	keep open
KP	keratoprecipitate; hot pack
KS	ketosteroids; Kaposi's sarcoma
17-KS	17-ketosteroids
KTU	kidney transplant unit
KUB	kidney, ureter, bladder
KVO	keep vein open
KW	Kimmelstiel-Wilson (disease); Keith-Wagener (ophthalmoscopic finding)
K-wire	Kirschner wire
L	left; liter; lumbar; lingual; lymphocyte; fifty
L2	second lumbar vertebra
LA	left atrium; local anesthesia; long acting; left arm; Latin American
L + A	light and accommodation
lab	laboratory
LAC	laceration; long arm cast
LAD	left anterior descending; left axis deviation
LAD-MIN	left axis deviation minimal
LAE	left atrial enlargement
LAF	lymphocyte-activating factor; laminar air flow; Latin American female
LAG	lymphangiogram
LAH	left atrial hypertrophy
LAL	left axillary line; limulus amebocyte lysate
LAM	Latin American male
LAN	lymphadenopathy
LAO	left anterior oblique
LAP	laparotomy; laparoscopy; left arterial pressure; leukocyte; leucine amino peptidase

LAPMS	long arm posterior molded splint	**LDA**	left dorsoanterior position
LAT	left anterior thigh; lateral	**LDB**	Legionnaires disease bacterium
LATS	long-acting thyroid stimulator	**LDDS**	local dentist
LAV	lymphadenopathy associated virus	**LDH**	lactic dehydrogenase
		LDL	low-density lipoprotein
LB	low back; left buttock; large bowel; left breast; pound	**LDP**	left dorsoposterior position
		LDV	laser Doppler velocimetry
LBB	left breast biopsy	**LE**	lupus erythematosus; lower extremities; left eye
LBBB	left bundle branch block		
LBCD	left border of cardiac dullness	**LED**	lupus erythematosus disseminatus
LBD	left border dullness		
LBF	Lactobacillus bulgaricus factor	**LEHPZ**	lower esophageal high pressure zone
LBD	left border dullness		
LBM	lean body mass; loose bowel movement	**L-ERX**	leukoerythroblastic reaction
		LES	lower esophageal sphincter; local excitatory state
LBO	large bowel obstruction		
LBP	low back pain; low blood pressure	**LESP**	lower esophageal sphincter pressure
LBT	lupus band test	**LET**	linear energy transfer
LBV	left brachial vein	**LF**	low forceps; left foot
LBW	low birth weight; lean body weight	**LFA**	left fronto-anterior; low friction arthroplasty
LC	living children; low calorie	**LFC**	living female child
LCA	left coronary artery; Leber's congenital amaurosis	**LFD**	low fat diet; low forceps delivery; lactose free diet
LCCA	leukocytoclastic angitis; left common carotid artery	**LFP**	left frontoposterior
		LFS	liver function studies
LCCS	low cervical Cesarean section	**LFT**	liver function test; left frontotransverse; latex flocculation test
LCD	liquor carbonis detergens (coal tar solution); localized collagen dystrophy		
		lg	large; left gluteus
LCGU	local cerebral glucose utilization	**LG**	lymph glands
		LGA	large for gestational age
LCH	local city hospital	**LGL**	Lown-Ganong-Levine (syndrome)
LCLC	large cell lung carcinoma		
LCM	left costal margin; lymphocytic choriomeningitis	**LGV**	lymphagranuloma venereum
		LH	luteinizing hormone; left hyperphoria; left hand
LCR	late cutaneous reaction		
LCS	low constant suction; low continuous suction	**LHF**	left heart failure
		LHL	left hemisphere lesions
LCT	long chain triglyceride; low cervical transverse; lymphocytotoxicity	**LHP**	left hemiparesis
		LHR	leukocyte histamine release
		LHRH	luteinizing hormone-releasing hormone
LCV	low cervical vertical		
LCX	left circumflex coronary artery	**LHT**	left hypertropia
LD	lethal dose; loading dose; liver disease; labor and delivery	**LIB**	left in bottle

LIC	left iliac crest; left internal carotid	**LN**	lymph nodes
LICA	left internal carotid artery	**LND**	lymph node dissection
LIF	left iliac fossa; liver inhibitory factor	**LNMP**	last normal menstrual period
lig	ligament	**LO**	lateral oblique
LIH	left inguinal hernia	**LOA**	left occiput anterior; leave of absence
LIMA	left internal mammary artery (graft)	**LOC**	loss of consciousness; level of consciousness; level of care; laxative of choice; local
LIP	lymphocytic interstitial pneumonia	**LOD**	line of duty
LIQ	lower inner quadrant; liquid	**LOM**	limitation of motion; left otitis media
LIS	low intermittent suction	**LoNa**	low sodium
LISREL	(computer program that performs structural equation modeling)	**LOP**	left occiput posterior; leave on pass
LISS	low ionic strength saline	**LOQ**	lower outer quadrant
LK	left kidney	**LORS**	Level of Rehabilitation Scale
LKKS	liver, kidneys, spleen	**LOS**	length of stay
LKS	liver, kidneys, spleen	**LOT**	left occiput transverse
LL	large lymphocyte; lumbar length; lymphoblastic lymphoma; left leg; lower lip	**LOV**	loss of vision
		loz	lozenge
LLB	long leg brace	**LP**	lumbar puncture; light perception
LLC	long leg case	**LPC**	laser photocoagulation
LLE	left lower extremity	**lpf**	low-power field
LL-GXT	low-level graded exercise test	**LPD**	luteal phase defect
LLL	left lower lobe; left lower lid	**LPF**	low power field
LLO	Legionella-like organism	**LPH**	left posterior hemiblock
LLQ	left lower quadrant	**LPO**	left posterior oblique; light perception only
LLS	lazy leukocyte syndrome	**LPP**	lipoprotein lipase
LLSB	left lower sternal border	**LR**	light reflex; labor room; left-right
LLT	left lateral thigh		
LMA	left mento-anterior; liver membrane autoantibody	**L>R**	left to right
		LRD	living renal donor
LMB	Laurence-Moon-Biedl syndrome	**LRND**	left radical neck dissection
		LRQ	lower right quadrant
LMC	living male child	**L-S**	lumbo-sacral
LMCA	left main coronary artery	**L/S**	lecithin-spingomyelin ratio
LMD	low molecular weight dextran	**LSA**	left sacrum anterior; lipid-bound sialic acid; lymphosarcoma
LMEE	left middle ear exploration		
L/min	liters per minute		
LML	left medial lateral/lobe	**LSB**	left sternal border
LMM	lentigo maligna melanoma	**LS BPS**	laparoscopic bilateral partial salpingectomy
LMP	last menstrual period; left mentoposterior		
		LSD	low salt diet
LMT	left mentotransverse	**LSE**	local side effects
LMWD	low molecular weight dextran	**LSF**	low saturated fat

260

LSKM	liver-spleen-kidney-megalia
LSM	late systolic murmur
LSO	left salpingo-oophorectomy
LSP	left sacrum posterior; liver-specific (membrane) lipoprotein
L/S ratio	lecithin/sphingomyelin ratio
LSS	liver-spleen scan
LST	left sacrum transverse
LSTL	laparoscopic tubal ligation
LT	light; left; left thigh; lumbar traction; levin tube; leukotrienes
LTB	laparoscopic tubal banding; laryngotracheo bronchitis
LTC	long-term care; left to count
LTCF	long-term care facility
LTCS	low transverse cesarean section
LTGA	left transposition of great artery
LTL	laparoscopic tubal ligation
LTT	lymphocyte transformation test
L & U	lower and upper
LUE	left upper extremity
LUL	left upper lobe
LUQ	left upper quadrant
LUSB	left upper sternal border
LV	left ventricle
LVA	left ventricular aneurysm
LVAD	left ventricular assist device
LVE	left ventricular enlargement
LVEDP	left ventricular end diastolic pressure
LVEDV	left ventricular end diastolic volume
LVEF	left ventricular ejection fraction
LVF	left ventricular failure
LVFP	left ventricular filling pressure
LVH	left ventricular hypertrophy
LVL	left vastus lateralis
LVMM	left ventricular muscle mass
LVP	left ventricular pressure; large volume parenteral
LVPW	left ventricular posterior wall

LVSWI	left ventricular stroke work index
LVV	left ventricular volume
L & W	living and well
LWCT	Lee-White clotting time
LYG	lymphmatoid granulomatosis
lymphs	lymphocytes
lytes	electrolytes
M	murmur; meter; minimum; medial; myopia; monocytes; male; molar; married; thousand
M_1	first mitral sound
M^2	square meters (body surface)
MA	mental age; medical assistance; milliamps; menstrual age; Miller-Abbott (tube)
M/A	mood and/or affect
MAA	macroaggregates of albumin
MAB	monoclonal antibody
MABP	mean arterial blood pressure
MAC	maximum allowable concentration; midarm circumference; minimum alveolar concentration; mycobacterium avium complex
MAE	moves all extremities
MAEEW	moves all extremities equally well
MAFAs	movement-associated fetal (heart rate) accelerations
MAHA	macroangiopathic hemolytic anemia
MAI	mycobacterium avium-intracellulare
MAL	midaxillary line
MALT	mucosa-associated lymphoid tissue
MAMC	mid-arm muscle circumference
mammo	mammography
MAOI	monoamine oxidase inhibitor
mand	mandibular

261

MAP	mean arterial pressure	MDC	medial dorsal cutaneous (nerve)
MAS	meconium aspiration syndrome; mobile arm support	MDD	manic depressive disorder; major depressive disorder
MAST	military antishock trousers	MDF	myocardial depressant factor
MAT	multifocal atrial tachycardia	MDI	multiple daily injection; metered dose inhaler
max	maximal; maxillary		
M-BACOD	a drug combination protocol	MDII	multiple daily insulin injection
MBC	maximum breathing capacity; minimal bacteriocidal concentration	MDM	middiastolic murmur; minor determinant mix
MB-CK	a creatinine kinase isoenzyme	MDR	minimum daily requirement
MBD	minimal brain damage; minimal brain dysfunction	MDS	maternal deprivation syndrome
		MDTP	multidisciplinary treatment plan
MBI	methylene blue installation	ME	macula edema; medical examiner; middle ear
MBM	mother's breast milk	MEA-I	multiple endocrine adenomatosis type I
MC	mixed cellularity; metatarso-cuneiform		
MCA	middle cerebral aneurysm; middle cerebral artery; motorcycle accident; monoclonal antibodies	mec	meconium
		MED	median erythrocyte diameter; medial; medical; medication; medicine; minimum erythema dose; medium
MCC	midstream clean-catch	MEDAC	multiple endocrine deficiency-autoimmune-candidiasis
MCCU	midstream clean-catch urine		
MCD	minimal change disease		
mcg	microgram	MEE	middle ear effusion
MCGN	minimal change glomerular nephritis	MEF	maximum expired flow rate
		MEFV	maximum expiratory flow-volume
MCH	mean corpuscular hemoglobin; muscle contraction headache	MEN (II)	multiple endocrine neoplasia (type II)
MCHC	mean corpuscular hemoglobin concentration	MEOS	microsomal ethanol oxidizing system
MCL	midclavicular line; midcostal line	mEq	milliequivalent
		M/E ratio	myeloid/erythroid ratio
MCLNS	mucocutaneous lymph node syndrome	META	metamyelocytes
		METS	metabolic equivalents (multiples of resting oxygen uptake); metastases
MCP	metacarpophalangeal joint		
MCS	microculture and sensitivity		
MCSA	minimal cross-sectional area		
MCT	medium chain triglyceride; mean circulation time	MF	myocardial fibrosis; mycosis fungoides; midcavity forceps
MCTD	mixed connective tissue disease	M & F	mother and father; male and female
MCV	mean corpuscular volume	MFA	mid-forceps delivery
MD	medical doctor; mental deficiency; muscular dystrophy; manic depression	MFAT	multifocal atrial tachycardia
		MFEM	maximal forced expiratory maneuver
MDA	manual dilation of the anus	MFH	malignant fibrous histiocytoma

MFR	mid-forceps rotation	MLC	mixed lymphocyte culture; minimal lethal concentraiton
MG	myasthenia gravis; milligram; Marcus Gunn	MLD	metachromatic leukodystrophy; minimal lethal dose
MGF	maternal grandfather		
MGM	maternal grandmother	MLF	median longitudinal fasiculus
MGN	membranous glomerulonephritis	MLNS	mucocutaneous lymph node syndrome
MGUS	monoclonal gammapathies of undetermined significance	MLR	mixed lymphocyte reaction
		MM	millimeter; mucous membrane; multiple myeloma
M-GXT	multi-stage graded exercise test	mM	millimole
MH	marital history; menstrual history; mental health; malignant hyperthermia	M & M	milk and molassses; morbidity and mortality
		MMECT	multiple monitor electroconvulsive therapy
MHA	microangiopathic hemolytic anemia	MMEFR	maximal midexpiratory flow rate
MHB	maximum hospital benefit	MMF	mean maximum flow
MHC	major histocompatibility complex; mental health center	MMFR	maximal midexpiratory flow rate
		mmHg	millimeters of mercury
MH/MR	mental health and mental retardation	MMK	Marshall-Marchetti-Krantz (cystourethropexy)
MI	myocardial infarction; mitral insufficiency; mental institution	MMOA	maxillary mandibular odentectomy alveolectomy
		mmol	millimole
MIA	medically indigent adult; missing in action	MMPI	Minnesota Multiphasic Personality Inventory
MIC	minimum inhibitory concentration; maternal and infant care	MMR	measles, mumps, rubella; midline malignant reticulosis
		MMS	Mini-Mental State (examination)
MICN	mobile intensive care nurse	MMT	manual muscle test
MICU	medical intensive care unit; mobile intensive care unit	MMWR	Morbidity & Mortality Weekly Report
MID	multi-infarct dementia	MN	midnight
MIDD	monoclonal immunoglobulin deposition	M & N	morning and night
		MNC	mononuclear leukocytes
MIF	migration inhibitory factor	MNG	multinodular goiter
MIH	migraine with interparoxysmal headache	MNR	marrow neutrophil reserve
		Mn SSEPS	median nerve somatosensory evoked potentials
min	minimum; minute; minor		
MIO	minimum identifiable odor	MNTB	medial nucleus of the trapezoid body
MIRP	myocardial infarction rehabilitation program		
mlx mon	mixed monitor	MO	month; medial oblique
MJT	Mead Johnson tube	MOA	mechanism of action
MKAB	may keep at bedside	MOB	medical office building
ML	midline; milliliter; middle lobe		
mL	milliliter		

MOD	medical officer of the day; moderate	**MSR**	muscle stretch reflexes
MODY	maturity onset diabetes of youth	**MSS**	minor surgery suite; muscular subaortic stenosis; Marital Satisfaction Scale
MOF	multiple organ failure	**MST**	mean survival time
mono	monocyte; infectious mononucleosis	**MSTA®**	mumps skin test antigen
		MSU	midstream urine
mOsm	milliosmole	**MSUD**	maple syrup urine disease
mOsmol	milliosmole	**MSW**	multiple stab wounds; Master of Social Work
MP	metacarpal phalangeal joint		
MPGN	membranoproliferative glomerulonephritis	**MT**	music therapy; medical technologist
MPH	Master of Public Health	**MTAL**	medullary thick ascending limb
MPJ	metacarpophalangeal joint	**MTD**	Monro Tidal drainage
MPL	maximum permissable level	**MTI**	malignant teratoma intermiate
MPS	mucopolysaccharidosis	**MTM**	modified Thayer-Martin medium
MPTR( )	motor, pain, touch reflex deficit		
MR	mental retardation; may repeat; magnetic resonance; mitral regurgitation	**MTP**	metatarsal phalangeal
		MTU	malignant teratoma undifferentiated
		MU	million units
MR x 1	may repeat times one	**MUDPIES**	methanol, uremia, diabetic ketoacidosis, paraldehyde, idiopathic, ethylene glycol, salicylate (cause of metabolic acidosis)
MRA	medical record administrator		
MRAN	medical resident admitting note		
MRD	Medical Records Department		
MRG	murmurs, rubs and gallops	**MULEPAK**	methanol, uremia, lactic acidosis, ethylene glycol, paraldehyde, aspirin, diabetic ketoacidosis (cause of metabolic acidosis)
MRI	magnetic resonance imaging		
mRNA	messenger ribonucleic acid		
MRS	magnetic resonance spectroscopy		
MRSA	methicillin resistant Staphylococcus aureus	**MUGA**	multiple gated acquisition
MS	multiple sclerosis; mitral stenosis; musculoskeletal; medical student; minimal support; muscle strength; mental status	**MUGX**	multiple gated acquisition exercise
		MVA	motor vehicle accident; malignant ventricular arrhythmias
M & S	microculture and sensitivity	**MVB**	mixed venous blood
MSAF	meconium stained amniotic fluid	**MVC**	maximal voluntary contraction
		MVI®	parenteral multivitamins
MSAFP	maternal serum alpha fetoprotein	**MVO₂**	myocardial oxygen consumption
MSC	medical social consultant	**MVP**	mitral valve prolapse
MSE	Mental Status Examination	**MVR**	mitral valve replacement; mitral valve regurgitation
MSH	melanocyte-stimulating hormone		
		MVS	mitral valve stenosis
MSK	medullary sponge kidney	**MVV**	maximum voluntary ventilation; mixed vespid venom
MSL	midsternal line		

MWS	Mickety-Wilson syndrome
My	myopia
myelo	myelocyte
N	normal; negative; Negro
5'-N	5'-Nucleotidase
NA	nursing assistant; nurse anesthetist; not applicable
NAA	neutron activation analysis
NABS	normoactive bowel sounds
NAD	no acute distress; no apparent distress; no appreciable disease; normal axis deviation; nothing abnormal detected
NAG	narrow angle glaucoma
NANB	non-A, non-B hepatitis
NAS	no added salt; neonatal abstinence syndrome
NAT	no action taken
NB	newborn; note well; needle biopsy
NBM	no bowel movement; normal bowel movement; nothing by mouth
NBN	newborn nursery
NBS	normal bowel sound; no bacteria seen
NBT	nitroblue tetrazolium reduction test
NBTE	nonbacterial thrombotic endocarditis
NC	neurologic check; no complaints; not completed; nasal cannula
NCA	neurocirculatory athenia
NC/AT	normal cephalic atraumatic
NCB	no code blue
NCD	normal childhood diseases; not considered disabling
NCF	neutrophilic chemotactic factor
NCI	National Cancer Institute
NCJ	needle catheter jejunostomy
NCL	neuronal ceroid lipofuscinosis
NCM	nailfold capillary microscopy
NCNC	normochromic, normocytic
NCPR	no cardiopulmonary resuscitation

NCS	no concentrated sweets; nerve conduction studies
NCV	nerve conduction velocity
ND	normal delivery; normal development; not done; not diagnosed; nasal deformity
NDA	new drug application
NDD	no dialysis days
NDT	neurodevelopmental treatment
NDV	Newcastle disease virus
NE	norepinephrine; not elevated; not examined
NEC	necrotizing entercolitis; not elsewhere classified
NED	no evidence of disease
NEG	negative
NEMD	nonsepcific esophageal motility disorder
NET	naso-endotracheal tube
neut	neutrophil
NF	negro female; not found; neurofibromatosis
NFL	nerve fiber layer
NFTD	normal full term delivery
NFTT	nonorganic failure to thrive
NFW	nursed fairly well
NG	nasogastric; nanogram
NGF	nerve growth factor
NGR	nasogastric replacement
NGT	nasogastric tube
NGU	nongonococcal urethritis
NH	nursing home
NHD	normal hair distribution
NHL	non-Hodgkin's lymphoma; nodular histocytic lymphoma
NHP	nursing home placement
NCC	neonatal intensive care center
NICU	neurosurgical intensive care unit; neonatal intensive care unit
NIDD	non-insulin-dependent diabetes
NIDDM	non-insulin-dependent diabetes mellitus
NIF	negative inspiratory force
NIH	National Institutes of Health
NINVS	non-invasive neurovascular studies

NJ	nasojejunal
NK	natural killer (cells)
NKA	no known allergies
NKDA	no known drug allergies
NKHS	nonketotic hyperosmolar syndrome
NKMA	no known medication allergies
NL	normal; normal limits
NLD	necrobiosis lipoidica diabeticorum; nasolacrimal duct
NLF	nasolabial fold
NLP	nodular liquifying panniculitis; no light perception
NLT	not later than; not less than
NM	negro male; neuromuscular; nodular melanoma
NMD	normal muscle development
NMR	nuclear magnetic resonance
NMI	no middle initial
NMS	neuroleptic malignant syndrome
NMT	no more than
NN	neonatal; nursing notes
NND	neonatal death
NNE	neonatal necrotizing enterocolitis
NNM	Nicole-Novy-MacNeal (media)
NNO	no new orders
NNP	neonatal nurse practitioner
NNU	net nitrogen utilization
no	number
noc	night
noct	nocturnal
NOD	notify of death
NOMI	nonocclusive mesenteric infarction
NOOB	not out of bed
NOS	not otherwise specified
NOSIE	Nurse Observation Scale for Inpatient Evaluation
NP	neuropsychiatric; nasopharyngeal; newly presented; no pain; not pregnant; not present; nursed poorly; nasal prongs
NPA	near point of accommodation
NPC	near point convergences; nodal premature contractions; nonpatient contact
NPDL	nodular poorly differentiated lymphocytic
NPDR	nonproliferative diabetic retinopathy
NPH	normal pressure hydrocephalis; no previous history
NPO	nothing by mouth
NPT	normal pressure and temperature; nocturnal penile tumescence
NR	nonreactive
NRBS	non-rebreathing system
NRC	normal retinal correspondence
NREM	nonrapid eye movement
NREMS	nonrapid eye movement sleep
NRT	neuromuscular reeducation techniques
NS	nephrotic syndrome; nuclear sclerosis; not seen; not significant; nylon suture
NSA	normal serum albumin; no significant abnormality
NSABP	National Surgical Adjuvant Breast Project
NSC	no significant change; not service connected
NSCLC	non-small-cell lung cancer
NSD	normal spontaneous delivery; nominal standard dose
NSDA	non-steroid dependent asthmatic
NSE	neuron-specific enolase
NSFTD	normal spontaneous full-term delivery
NSG	nursing
NSILA	nonsuppressible insulin-like activity
NSN	nephrotoxic serum nephritis
NSPVT	nonsustained polymorphic ventricular tachycardia
NSR	normal sinus rhythm; not seen regularly; nonspecific reaction; nasoseptal repair

NSSTT	nonspecific ST and T wave
NST	nutritional support team; non-stress test; not sooner than
NSU	nonspecific urethritis
NSV	nonspecific vaginitis
NSVD	normal spontaneous vaginal delivery
NT	not tested; nasotracheal; not tender
N & T	nose and throat
NTC	neurotrauma center
NTE	not to exceed
NTF	normal throat flora
NTG	nontreatment group
NTMB	nontuberculous myobacteria
NTMI	non-transmural myocardial infarction
NTP	normal temperature and pressure
NTS	nasotracheal suction; nucleus tractus solitarii
NTT	nasotracheal tube
NUD	nonulcer dyspepsia
nullip	nullipara
NV	neurovascular
N & V	nausea and vomiting
NVD	nausea, vomiting, and diarrhea; neck vein distention; no venereal disease; neurovesicle dysfunction; nonvalvular disease; neovascularization of the disc
NVE	neovascularization elsewhere
NVG	neovascular glaucoma
NVS	neurological vital signs
NWB	non-weight bearing
NYD	not yet diagnosed
NZ	enzyme
O	oxygen; objective finding; eye; oral; open; obvious; often; other; occlusal
1O$_2$	singlet oxygen
O$_2$	oxygen; both eyes
O$_2$v	superoxide

OA	oral alimentation; occiput anterior; osteoarthritis; Overeaters Anonymous
O & A	observation and assessment
OAF	osteoclast activating factor
Ob	obstetrics
OB	occult blood
OBE-CALP	placebo capsule or tablet
Ob-Gyn	obstetrics and gynecology
OBS	organic brain syndrome
OC	oral contraceptive; obstetrical conjugate; oral care; on call; office call
OCA	oculocutaneous albinism
OCCC	open chest cardiac compression
OCCM	open chest cardiac massage
OCG	oral cholecystogram
OCP	ova, cysts, parasites
OCT	oxytocin challenge test
OCU	observation care unit
OD	right eye; overdose; on duty; doctor of optometry
OER	oxygen enhancement ratios
OFC	occipital-frontal circumference
OG	orogastric (feeding)
OGTT	oral glucose tolerance test
OH	occupational history; open heart
OHA	oral hypoglycemic agents
OHD	organic heart disease
OHF	omsk hemorrhage fever
OHG	oral hypoglycemic
OHP	oxygen under hyperbaric pressure
OHRR	open heart recovery room
OHS	open heart surgery
OI	osteogenesis imperfecta
OIF	oil-immersion field
OJ	orthoplast jacket; orange juice
OKAN	optokinetic after nystagmus
OKN	optokinetic nystagmus
OLA	occiput left anterior
OM	otitis media; every morning
OME	Office of the Medical Examiner; otitis media with effusion
OMI	old myocardial infarct

OMR	operative mortality rate	P	plan; protein; pint; pulse; peripheral; phosphorous; para
OMSC	otitis media secretory/suppurative chronic	p	after
ON	overnight; every night	P_2	pulmonic second heart sound
ONC	over-the-needle catheter	PA	posterior-anterior; pulmonary artery; pernicious anemia; physician assistant; presents again; psychiatric aide; professional association
OOB	out of bed		
OOBBRP	out of bed with bathroom privileges		
OOC	out of control		
OOP	out on pass; out of pelvis		
OOR	out of room	P & A	percussion and auscultation
OOT	out of town	PAB	premature atrial beat
OP	outpatient; operation; occiput posterior; open	PAC	premature atrial contraction
		PACH	pipers to after coming head
O & P	ova and parasites	PADP	pulmonary artery diastolic pressure
OPB	outpatient basis		
OPC	outpatient clinic	PAF	paroxysmal atrial fibrillation; platelet activating factors
OPCA	olivopontocerebellar atrophy		
OPD	outpatient department	PAO_2	arterial oxygen tension
OPG	ocular plethysmography	$PaCO_2$	arterial carbon dioxide tension
OPM	occult primary malignancy	PAGE	polyacrylamide gel electrophoresis
OPPG	oculopneumoplethysmography		
OPS	operations	PAIVS	pulmonary atresia with intact ventricle septum
OPV	oral polio vaccine		
OR	operating room; oil retention	Pa Line	pulmonary artery line
ORIF	open reduction internal fixation	PALN	para-aortic lymph node
ORL	otorhinolaryngology	PAN	periodic alternating nystagmus; polyarteritis nodosa
OS	left eye; mouth; opening snap		
OSA	obstructive sleep apnea		
OSD	overside drainage	PAOP	pulmonary artery occlusion pressure
OSM S	osmolarity serum		
OSM U	osmolarity urine	PAP	pulmonary artery pressure; prostatic acid phosphatase
OSN	off service note		
OSS	osseous	Pap smear	Papanicolaou smear
OT	old tuberculin; occupational therapy	PA/PS	pulmonary atresia/pulmonary stenosis
OTC	over-the-counter	PAR	postanesthetic recovery; platelet aggregate ratio
OTD	out the door		
OTO	otology	PARA	number of pregnancies
OTR	Occupational Therapist, Registered	para	paraplegic
		PARU	postanesthetic recovery unit
OTS	orotracheal suction	PAS	periodic acid-Schiff (reagent); peripheral anterior synechia; pulmonary artery stenosis
OTT	orotracheal tube		
OU	both eyes		
OV	office visit; ovum; ovary	PasEx	passive exercise
OW	out of wedlock	PAT	paroxysmal atrial tachycardia; preadmission testing; percent acceleration time
oz	ounce		

Path	pathology
PAWP	pulmonary artery wedge pressure
Pb	lead
PB	powder board; parafin bath
PBA	percutaneous bladder aspiration
PBC	point of basal convergence; primary biliary cirrhosis
PBD	percutaneous biliary drainage
PBL	peripheral blood lymphocyte
PBMC	peripheral blood mononuclear cell
PBMNC	peripheral blood mononuclear cell
PBO	placebo
PC	after meal; packed cells; professional corporation; platelet concentrate
PCA	patient care assistant/aide; patient controlled analgesia; posterior cerebral artery; procoagulation activity; passive cutaneous anaphylaxis
PCCU	post coronary care unit
PCG	phonocardiogram
PCH	paroxysmal cold hemoglobinuria
PCI	prophylactic cranial irradiation
PCIOL	posterior chamber intraocular lens
PCL	posterior chamber lens; posterior cruciate ligament
PCM	protein-calorie malnutrition
PCO	polycystic ovary
PCO$_2$	carbon dioxide pressure/tension
PCOD	polycystic ovarian disease
PCP	pneumonocystis carinii pneumonia; pulmonary capillary pressure
PCR	protein catabolic/caloric rate
PCT	porphyria cutanea
PCTA	percutaneous transluminal angioplasty
PCU	progressive care unit
PCV	packed cell volume

PCWP	pulmonary capillary wedge pressure
PD	peritoneal dialysis; postural drainage; Parkinson's disease; interpupillary distance; percutaneous drain
P/D	packs per day (cigarettes)
PDA	patent ductus arteriosus
PDE	paroxysmal dyspnea on exertion; pulsed Doppler echocardiography
PDFC	premature dead female child
PDGF	platelet derived growth factor
PDL	poorly differentiated lymphocytic
PDL-D	poorly differentiated lymphocytic-diffuse
PDL-N	poorly differentiated lymphocytic-nodular
PDMC	premature dead male child
PDN	private duty nurse
PDR	proliferative diabetic retinopathy; Physician's Desk Reference
PDS	pain dysfunction syndrome
PDGXT	predischarge graded exercise test
PDT	photodynamic therapy
PDU	pulsed Doppler ultrasonography
PE	physical examination; pulmonary embolism; pressure equalization; pleural effusion
PECHO	prostatic echogram
PECO$_2$	mixed expired carbon dioxide tension
Peds	pediatrics
PEEP	positive end-expiratory pressure
PEFR	peak expiratory flow rate
PEG	pneumoencephalogram; percutaneous endoscopic gastrostomy
PEN	parenteral and enteral nutrition
PENS	percutaneous epidural nerve stimulator

PEP	protein electrophoresis; pre-ejection period; Parkinson's educational program
PER	pediatric emergency room
perf	perforation
PERL	pupils equal, reactive to light
per os	by mouth
PERR	pattern evoked retinal response
PERRLA	pupils equal, round, reactive to light and accommodation
PES	pre-excitation syndrome
PET	positron-emission tomography; pre-eclamptic toxemia; pressure equalizing tubes
PF	power factor
PFC	persistent fetal circulation
PFM	porcelain fused to metal
PFR	peak flow rate; parotid flow rate
PFT	pulmonary function test
PFU	plaque-forming unit
PG	pregnant
PGF	parenteral grandfather
PGH	pituitary growth hormones
PGL	persistent generalized lymphadenopathy
PGM	paternal grandmother
PgR	progesterone receptor
PGU	postgonococcal urethritis
pH	hydrogen ion concentration
PH	past history; poor health; public health
PHA	passive hemagglutinating; phytohemagglutinin; arterial pH; phytohemagglutinin antigen; peripheral hyperalimentation
Pharm	pharmacy
PHC	primary hepatocellular carcinoma
PHH	posthemorrhagic hydrocephalus
PHN	public health nurse; post herpetic neuralgia
PHPT	primary hyperparathyroidism

PHPV	persistent hyperplastic primary vitreous
Phx	pharynx
PI	present illness; pulmonary infarction; peripheral iridectomy
PIAT	Peabody Individual Achievement Test
PICA	posterior inferior communicating artery; posterior inferior cerebellar artery
PICU	pediatric intensive care unit
PID	pelvic inflammatory disease; prolapsed intervertebral disc
PIE	pulmonary infiltration with eosinophilia; pulmonary interstitial emphysema
PIH	pregnancy induced hypertension
PISA	phase invariant signature alogrithm
PIOK	poikilocytosis
PIP	proximal interphalangeal joint; post inspiratiory pressure
PITR	plasma iron turnover rate
PIV	peripheral intravenous
PIVD	protruded intervertebral disc
PJB	premature junctional beat
PJC	premature junctional contractions
PJS	Peutz-Jeghers syndrome
PK	penetrating keratoplasty
PKD	polycystic kidney disease
PK test	Prausnitz-Kunstner transfer test
PKU	phenylketonuria
PL	plantar; place; light perception
PLAP	placental alkaline phosphatase
PLFC	premature living female child
PLH	paroxysmal localized hyperhidrosis
PLL	prolymphocytic leukemia
PLMC	premature living male child
PLN	pelvic lymph node; popliteal lymph node
PLS	primary lateral sclerosis
plts	platelets

PM	post mortem; evening; pretibial myxedema; primary motivation; presents mainly
PMA	Prinzmetal's angina; premenstrual asthma
PMB	postmenopausal bleeding; polymorphonuclear basophils
PMC	pseudomembranous colitis
PMD	private medical doctor
PME	post menopausal estrogen
PMF	progressive massive fibrosis
PMH	past medical history
PMI	point of maximal impulse; patient medication instructions
PML	progressive multifocal leukoencephalopathy
PMN	polymorphonuclear cell
PMP	pain management program; previous menstrual period
PMR	polymyalgia rheumatica; polymorphic reticulosis
PM & R	physical medicine and rehabilitation
PMS	premenstrual syndrome
PMT	premenstrual tension
PMTS	premenstrual tension syndrome
PMV	prolapse of mitral valve
PMW	pacemaker wires
PN	parenteral nutrition; progress note; percussion note
PNAS	prudent no salt added
PNB	premature nodal beat
PNC	premature nodal contraction; peripheral nerve conduction
PND	paroxysmal nocturnal dyspnea; postnasal drip
PNET-MB	primitive neuroectodermal tumors-medulloblastoma
PNF	proprioceptive neuromuscular fasiculation reaction
PNH	paroxysmal nocturnal hemoglobinuria
PNI	prognostic nutrition index; peripheral nerve injury
PNMG	persistent neonatal myasthenia gravis

PNP	Pediatric Nurse Practitioner; progressive nuclear palsy
PNS	peripheral nervous system; partial nonprogressing stroke; practical nursing student
PNT	percutaneous nephrostomy tube
PNU	protein nitrogen units
PNV	prenatal vitamins
Pnx	pneumothorax
PO	postoperative; phone order; by mouth (per os)
PO_2	partial pressure of oxygen
POA	pancreatic oncofetal antigen
POAG	primary open-angle glaucoma
POC	product of conception; postoperative care
POD 1	postoperative day one
POEMS	plasma cell dyscrasia with polyneuropathy, organomegaly, endocrinopathy, monoclonal (M)-protein, skin changes
POIK	poikilocytosis
POL	premature onset of labor
POLY	polymorphonuclear leukocyte
POMR	problem-oriented medical record
poplit	popliteal
PORT	postoperative respiratory therapy
POS	parosteal osteosarcoma
post	post mortem examination (autopsy)
post op	postoperative
PP	postpartum; postprandial; paradoxical pulse; pin prick; patient profile; protoporphyria; proximal phalynx; private patient; near point of accommodation
P & P	pins and plater
PPB	parts per billion
PPBG	postprandial blood glucose
PPBS	post prandial blood sugar
PPC	progressive patient care

PPD	packs per day; postpartum day; posterior polymorphous dystrophy	prep	prepare for surgery
		PRG	phleborrheogram
P & PD	percussion and postural drainage	PRIMP	primipara (first pregnancy)
		PRN	as needed
		PRO	protein
PPD-B	purified protein derivative, Battey	prob	probable
		PROC-TO	proctology; procotoscopic
PPD-S	purified protein derivative, standard	prog	prognosis; prognathism
		PROM	passive range of motion; premature rupture of membranes
PPF	plasma protein fraction		
PPG	photoplethysmography		
PPH	postpartum hemorrhage	ProMACE	a drug protocol combination
PPHN	persistent pulmonary hypertension of the newborn	prov	provisional
		PRP	panretinal photocoagulation
PPI	patient package insert	PRRE	pupils round, regular, equal
PPL	pars planus lensectomy	PRSs	positive rolandic spikes
PPLO	pleuro-pneumonia-like organisms	PRTH-C	prothrombin time control
		PRV	polycythemia rubra vera
PPM	parts per million	PRVEP	pattern reversal visual evoked potentials
PPN	peripheral parenteral nutrition		
PPNG	penicillinase producing Neisseria gonorrhoeae	PRW	polymerized ragweed
		PS	pulmonary stenosis; paradoxic sleep; pathologic stage; plastic surgery; serum from pregnant women; performance status
PPO	preferred provider organization		
PPP	postpartum psychosis		
PPPG	post prandial plasma glucose		
PPPBL	peripheral pulses palpable both legs		
		P & S	paracentesis and suction; pain and suffering
PPROM	prolonged premature rupture of membranes		
		PsA	psoriatic arthritis
PPS	postpartum sterilization; pneumococcal polysaccharide (vaccine)	PS I	healthy patient with localized pathological process
		PS II	patient with mild to moderate systemic disease
PPTL	postpartum tubal ligation		
PPVT	Peabody Picture Vocabulary Test	PS III	patient with severe systemic disease limiting activity, but not incapacitating
PR	per rectum; pulse rate; profile; Puerto Rican; far point of accommodation		
		PS IV	patient with incapacitating systemic disease
		PS V	moribund patient not expected to live
P & R	pulse and respiration; pelvic and rectal		
		PsA	psoriatic arthritis
PRA	plasma renin activity	PSC	posterior subcapsular cataract; primary sclerosing cholangitis
PRAT	platelet radioactive antiglobulin test		
PRBC	packed red blood cells		
PRCA	pure red cell aplasia	PSE	portal systemic encephalopathy
PRE	progressive/passive resistive exercise		
pre-op	before surgery	PSF	posterior spinal fusion

PSGN	post streptococcal glomerulonephritis		**PTPM**	posttraumatic progressive myelopathy
PSH	post spinal headache		**PTPN**	peripheral (vein) total parenteral nutrition
PSI	pounds per square inch			
PSM	presystolic murmur		**PTS**	prior to surgery
PSP	pancreatic spasmolytic peptide; progressive supranuclear palsy		**PTSD**	post-traumatic stress disorder
			PTT	partial thromboplastin time
			PTX	pneumothorax
PSRBOW	premature spontaneous rupture of bag of waters		**PU**	peptic ulcer; pregnancy urine
			PUD	peptic ulcer disease
PSS	progressive systemic sclerosis; physiologic saline solution		**PUFA**	polyunsaturated fatty acids
			pul	pulmonary
PSW	psychiatric social worker		**PUN**	plasma urea nitrogen
PSVT	paroxysmal supraventricular tachycardia		**PUO**	pyrexia of undetermined origin
			PUVA	psoralen-ultraviolet light
PT	physical therapy/therapist; patient; prothrombin time; pine tar; posterior tibial; pint;		**PV**	polycythemia vera; polio vaccine; portal vein; pulmonary vein; per vagina
PTA	prior to admission; plasma thromboplatin antecedent; pretreatment anxiety; pure-tone average; physical therapy assistant; percutaneous transluminal angioplasty		**P & V**	pyloroplasty and vagotomy
			PVB	premature ventricular beat
			PVC	premature ventricular contraction; pulmonary venous congestion
			PVD	patient very disturbed; peripheral vascular disease; posterior vitreous detachment
PTB	patellar tendon bearing			
PTBD-EF	percutaneous transhepatic biliary drainage-enteric feeding		**PVE**	premature ventricular extrasystole; perivenous encephalomyelitis
PTC	plasma thromboplastin components; percutaneous transhepatic cholangiography		**PVO**	peripheral vascular occlusion; pulmonary venous occlusion
PTCA	percutaneous transluminal coronary angioplasty		**PVOD**	pulmonary vascular obstructive disease
PTD	period to discharge; permanent and total disability		**PVP**	peripheral venous pressure
			PVR	peripheral vascular resistance; postvoiding residual; proliferative vitreoretinopathy; pulse-volume recording
PTE	proximal tibial epiphysis; pulmonary thromboembolism; pretibial edema			
			PVS	peritoneovenous shunt; pulmonic valve stenosis; percussion, vibration and suction
PTF	plasma thromboplastin factor			
PTH	post transfusion hepatitis; parathyroid hormone			
PTL	pre-term labor		**PVT**	paroxysmal ventricular tachycardia; private
PTMDF	pupils, tension, media, disc, fundus			
			PWB	partial weight bearing
pTNM	postsurgical resection-pathologic staging of cancer		**PWLV**	posterior wall of left ventricle

PWM	pokeweed mitogens
PWLV	posterior wall of left ventricle
PWP	pulmonary wedge pressure
PWV	polistes wasp venom
Px	physical exam; prognosis; pneumothorax; practice
PXE	pseudoxanthoma elasticum
PTx	parathyroidectomy
PY	pack years
q	every
QA	quality assurance
QAM	every morning
QCA	quantitative coronary angiography
qd	every day
q4h	every four hours
qh	every hour
qhs	every night
qid	four times daily
qn	every night
qns	quantity not sufficient
qod	every other day
qoh	every other hour
qon	every other night
qpm	every evening
QRS	principal deflection in an electrocardiogram
QS	sufficient quantity; every shift
QUART	quadrantectomy, axillary dissection and radiotherapy
qwk	once a week
R	respiration; right; rectum; regular; rate; regular insulin
RA	rheumatoid arthritis; right atrium; right auricle; right arm; room air
RABG	room air blood gas
RAC	right atrial catheter
RAD	right axis deviation; radical
RAE	right atrial enlargement
RAEB	refractory anemia, erythroblastic
RAG	room air gas
RAIU	radioactive iodine uptake
RALT	routine admission laboratory tests

RAM	rapid alternating movements
RAN	resident admission notes
RAO	right anterior oblique
RAP	right atrial pressure
RAPD	relative afferent pupillary defect
RAS	renal artery stenosis
RAST	radioallergosorbent test
RAT	right anterior thigh
RA test	test for rheumatoid factor
R(AW)	airway resistance
RB	retrobulbar; right buttock
R & B	right and below
RBA	right brachial artery
RBB	right breast biopsy
RBBB	right bundle branch block
RBCD	right border cardiac dullness
RBC	red blood cell/count
RBD	right border of dullness
RBE	relative biologic effectiveness
RBF	renal blood flow
RBOW	rupture bag of water
RBP	retinol-binding protein
RBV	right brachial vein
R/C	reclining chair
RCA	right coronary artery; radionuclide cerebral angiogram; regional citrate anticoagulation
RCC	renal cell carcinoma
RCD	relative cardiac dullness
RCM	right costal margin; radiographic contrast media
RCS	reticulum cell sarcoma
RCT	root canal therapy
RCV	red cell volume
RD	registered dietitian; renal disease; retinal detachment; respiratory disease
RDA	recommended daily allowance
RDPE	reticular degeneration of pigment epithelium
RDH	Registered Dental Hygienist
RDS	respiratory distress syndrome
RDT	regular dialysis/hemodialysis treatment
RDVT	recurrent deep vein thrombosis

RE	reticuloendothelial; rectal examination; regional enteritis; right eye; concerning	**RICU**	respiratory intensive care unit
		RID	radial immunodiffusion
		RIF	rigid internal fixation; right iliac fossa
REE	resting energy expenditure	**RIH**	right inguinal hernia
REF	renal erythropoietic factor; referred	**RIMA**	right internal mammary anastamosis
rehab	rehabilitation	**RIND**	reversible ischemic neurologic defect
Rel	religion		
REM	rapid eye movement	**RIP**	radioimmunoprecipitin test; rapid infusion pump
REMS	rapid eye movement sleep		
REP	repeat; report; repair	**RISA**	radioactive iodinated serum albumin
repol	repolarization		
RER	renal excretion rate	**RIST**	radioimmunosorbent test
RES	reticuloendothelial system; resident	**RK**	radial keratotomy
		RL	right leg; right lung; right lateral
RESC	resuscitation	**R-L**	right to left
resp	respiratory; respiration	**RLE**	right lower extremity
retic	reticulocyte	**RLF**	retrolental fibroplasia
REV	revolutions; review; reverse	**RLL**	right lower lobe
RF	rheumatoid factor; rheumatic fever; renal failure	**RLQ**	right lower quadrant
		RLR	right lateral rectus
RFA	right fronto-anterior; right femoral artery	**RLT**	right lateral thigh
		RM	repetitions maximum; room; radical mastectomy; respiratory movement
RFL	right frontolateral		
RFP	right frontoposterior		
RFT	right frontotransverse	**R & M**	routine and microscopic
RG	right gluteal	**RMA**	right meno-anterior
RGM	right gluteus medius	**RMCA**	right main coronary artery
Rh	Rhesus factor in blood	**RMCL**	right midclavicular line
RH	right hyperphoria; right hand; reduced haloperidol; room humidifier	**RMD**	rapid movement disorder
		RME	right mediolateral episiotomy
		RMEE	right middle ear exploration
RHB	raise head of bed	**RML**	right middle lobe
RHC	respiration has ceased	**RMP**	right mentoposterior
RHD	rheumatic heart disease; relative hepatic dullness	**RMR**	right medial rectus; resting metabolic rate
RHE	recombinant human erythropoietin	**RMSF**	Rocky Mountain spotted fever
		RMT	right mentotransverse; registered music therapist
RHF	right heart failure		
RHL	right hemisphere lesions	**RN**	registered nurse
R-HuEPO	recombinant human erythropoietin	**RNA**	radionuclide angiography
		RND	radial neck dissection
RHT	right hypertropia	**RNEF**	resting/radio nuclide ejection fraction
RIA	radioimmunoassay		
RIC	right iliac crest; right internal carotid (artery)	**RO**	rule out; routine order
		ROA	right occiput anterior
RICS	right intercostal space	**ROM**	range of motion

275

ROP	right occiput posterior; retinopathy of prematurity	**RRND**	right radical neck dissection
ROS	review of systems	**RRR**	regular rhythm and rate
ROSC	restoration of spontaneous circulation	**RRRN**	round, regular, react normally
		RS	Reiter's syndrome; Reye's syndrome; rhythm strip; right side
RoRx	radiation therapy		
ROT	right occipital transverse; remedial occupational therapy	**RSA**	right sacrum anterior; right subclavian artery
RQ	respiratory quotient	**RSDS**	reflex-sympathetic dystrophy syndrome
RP	retinitis pigmentosa; retrograde pyelogram; Raynaud's phenomenon	**R-SICU**	respiratory-surgical intensive care unit
RPA	right pulmonary artery; radial photon absorptiometry; registered physician assistant/associate	**RSO**	right salpingo-oophorectomy; radiation safety officer
		RSP	right sacroposterior
		RSR	regular sinus rhythm; relative survival rate
RPCF	Reiter protein complement fixation	**RSTs**	Rodney Smith tubes
RPD	removable partial denture	**RSV**	respiratory syncytial virus
RPE	retinal pigment epithelium; rating of perceived exertion	**RSW**	right-sided weakness
		RT	right; radiation therapy; recreational therapy; renal transplant; running total; respiratory therapist
RPF	renal plasma flow; relaxed pelvic floor		
RPGN	rapidly progressive glomerulonephritis		
		R/t	related to
RPH	retroperitoneal hemorrhage; registered pharmacist	**RTA**	renal tubular acidosis
		RTC	return to clinic; round the clock
RPICCE	round pupil intracapsular cataract extraction	**RTL**	reactive to light
		RTM	routine medical care
RPLND	retroperitoneal lymphadenectomy	**rTNM**	retreatment staging of cancer
		RTO	return to office
RPM	renal parenchymal malacoplakia	**RTOG**	Radiation Therapy Oncology Group
RPN	renal papillary necrosis		
RPO	right posterior oblique	**rtPA**	recombinant tissue-type plasminogen
RPP	rate-pressure product		
RPR	rapid plasma reagin; Reiter protein reagin	**RTRR**	return to recovery room
		RTS	real time scan
RPT	registered physical therapist	**RT3U**	resin triiodothyronine uptake
RQ	respiratory quotient	**RTx**	radiation therapy
RR	recovery room; respiratory rate; regular respirations	**RUA**	routine urine analysis
		RUE	right upper extremity
R & R	rate and rhythm	**RUG**	retrograde urethrogram
RRE	round, regular and equal	**RUL**	right upper lobe
RREF	resting radionuclide ejection fraction	**rupt**	ruptured
		RUQ	right upper quadrant
		RURTI	recurrent upper respiratory tract infection
rRNA	ribosomal ribonucleic acid	**RUSB**	right upper sternal border

RV	right ventricle; residual volume; rectovaginal; rubella vaccine	**SAPD**	self-administration of psychotropic drugs
RVD	relative vertebral density	**SAS**	sleep apnea syndrome
RVE	right ventricular enlargement	**SAT**	subacute thyroiditis; saturation
RVET	right ventricular ejection time	**SAVD**	spontaneous assisted vaginal delivery
RVG	radionuclide ventriculography	**SB**	stillbirth; stillborn; spina bifida; sternal border; Sengstaken Blakemore (tube); sinus bradycardia; small bowel
RVH	right ventricular hypertrophy; renovascular hypertension		
RVL	right vastus lateralis		
RVO	retinal vein occlusion; relaxed vaginal outlet	**SBE**	subacute bacterial endocarditis
RVOT	right ventricular outflow tract	**SBFT**	small bowel follow through
RVR	rapid ventricular response	**SBGM**	self blood glucose monitoring
RVSWI	right ventricular stroke work index	**SBI**	systemic bacterial infection
		SB-LM	Stanford Binet Intelligence Test-Form LM
RV/TLC	residual volume to total lung capacity ratio	**SBO**	small bowel obstruction
RVV	rubella vaccine virus	**SBP**	systolic blood pressure; spontaneous bacterial peritonitis
Rx	therapy; drug; medication; treatment; take		
RXN	reaction	**SBR**	strict bed rest
		SBT	serum bacterial titers
S	subjective findings; serum; suction; sacral; single; sister	**SC**	subcutaneous; subclavian; sternoclavicular; sickle-cell; sulfur colloid; service connected
S_1	first heart sound; sacral vertebrae 1		
S_2	second heart sound	**SCA**	subcutaneous abdominal (block)
SA	sinoatrial; salicylic acid; sustained action; surface area; Spanish American		
		SCB	strictly confined to bed
		SCBC	small cell bronchogenic carcinoma
S/A	sugar and acetone		
SAB	subarachnoid block/bleed	**SCC**	squamous cell carcinoma; sickle cell crisis
SAC	short arm cast		
SACH	solid ankle cushion heel	**SCCa**	squamous cell carcinoma
SAD	sugar and acetone determination	**SCCA**	semi-closed circle absorber
		SCD	sudden cardiac death; sickle cell disease; subacute combined degeneration; service connected disability; spinal cord disease
SAF	self-articulating femoral		
Sag D	sagittal diameter		
SAH	subarachnoid hemorrhage; systemic arterial hypertension		
		SCE	sister chromatid exchange
SAL 12	sequential analysis of 12 chemistry constituents	**SCI**	spinal cord injury
		SCID	severe combined immunodeficiency disorder
SAM	systolic anterior motion; self-administered medication		
		SCIV	subclavian intravenous
SAN	sinoatrial node	**SCLC**	small-cell lung cancer
sang	sanguinous	**SCLE**	subcutaneous lupus erythematosis

SCLs	soft contact lenses	**SFA**	superficial femoral artery; saturated fatty acids
SCM	sternocleidomastoid; spondylitic caudal myelopathy	**SFC**	spinal fluid count
		SFEMG	single-fiber electromyography
SCR	spondylitic caudal radioculopathy	**SFP**	spinal fluid pressure
		SFPT	standard fixation preference test
SCT	sickle cell trait; sugar coated tablet	**SG**	specific gravity; serum glucose; Swan-Ganz
SCUT	schizophrenia chronic undifferentiated type	**SGA**	small for gestational age
		SGD	straight gravity drainage
SCV	subcutaneous vaginal (block)	**SGE**	significant glandular enlargement
SD	senile demenita; scleroderma; spontaneous delivery; sterile dressing; surgical drain	**s gl**	without correction/glasses
		SGOT	serum glutamic oxaloacetic transaminase
S & D	stomach and duodenum	**SGPT**	serum glutamic pyruvic transaminase
SDA	steroid-dependent asthmatic; Seventh-Day Adventist	**SH**	serum hepatitis; social history; shower; short; shoulder
SDAT	senile dementia of Alzheimer's type	**S & H**	speech and hearing
SDH	subdural hematoma	**S/H**	suicidal/homicidal ideation
SDL	serum digoxin level	**SHA**	super heater aerosol
SDS	same day surgery	**S Hb**	sickle hemoglobin screen
SDT	Speech Detection Threshold	**SHEENT**	skin, head, eyes, ears, nose throat
SE	side effect		
sec	secondary	**SHS**	Student Health Service
sed	sedimentation	**SI**	sacroiliac
sed rt	sedimentation rate	**SIADH**	system of inappropriate antidiuretic hormone secretion
SEER	Surveillance, Epidemiology, and End Results (program)		
seg	segment; segmented neutrophil	**S & I**	suction and irrigation
		SIB	self-injurious behavior
SEM	systolic ejection murmur; scanning electron microscopy; standard error of mean	**sibs**	siblings
		SICT	selective intracoronary thrombolysis
SEMI	subendocardial myocardial infarction	**SICU**	surgical intensive care unit
		SIDS	sudden infant death syndrome
SENS	sensorium	**sig**	let it be marked
SEP	systolic ejection period; somatosensory evoked potential; separate	**SIJ**	sacroiliac joint
		SIMV	synchronized intermittent mandatory ventilation
SER-IV	supination external rotation, type 4 fracture	**SIT**	sperm immobilization test; Slossen Intelligence Test
SERs	somatosensory evoked responses	**SIW**	self-inflicted wound
SES	socioeconomic status	**SJS**	Stevens-Johnson syndrome
SF	scarlet fever; sugar free; salt free; symptom free; spinal fluid	**SK**	SmithKline®
		SL	sublingual; slight

SLB	short leg brace	SOB	shortness of breath
SLC	short leg cast	S & OC	signed and on chart (permission)
SLE	systemic lupus erythematosus; slit lamp examination	SOD	surgical officer of the day; superoxide dysmutase
SLGXT	symptom limited graded exercise test	sol	solution
SLK	superior limbic keratoconjunctivitis	SOM	serous otitis media
		SOMI	sterno-occipital mandibular immobilizer
SLR	straight leg raising	Sono	sonogram
SLRT	straight leg raising cast	SONP	solid organs not palpable
SLWC	short leg walking cast	SOP	standard operating procedure
SM	systolic murmur; small	SOS	may be repeated once if urgently required
SMA	sequential multiple analyzer; simultaneous multichannel autoanalyzer; superior mesenteric artery; spinal muscular atrophy	SOT	stream of thought
		SP	suprapubic; sequential pulse; sacrum to pubis; speech pathologist
SMC	special mouth care		
SMD	senile macular degeneration	S/P	status post
SMI	small volume infusion; sustained maximal inspiration	SPA	albumin human; stimulation produced analgesia
SMON	subacute myeloopticoneuropathy	SPAG	small particle aerosol generator
SMP	self-management program	SPBI	serum protein bound iodine
SMR	submucosal resection; standardized mortality ratio; skeletal muscle relaxant; senior medical resident	SPBT	suprapubic bladder tap
		SPE	serum protein electrolytes
		spec	specimen
		SPECT	single photon emission computer tomography
SMS	senior medical student	Spec Ed	special education
SMVT	sustained monomorphic ventricular tachycardia	SPEP	serum protein electrophoresis
SN	student nurse	SPF	sun protective factor
SNAP	sensory nerve action potential	sp fl	spinal fluid
SNCV	sensory nerve conduction velocity	sp gr	specific gravity
		SPK	superficial punctate keratitis
SND	sinus node dysfunction	SPMA	spinal progressive muscle atrophy
SNE	subacute necrotizing encephalomyelopathy	SPMSQ	Short Portable Mental Status Questionnaire
SNF	skilled nursing facility		
SNGFR	single nephron glomerular filtration rate	SPN	solitary pulmonary nodule
		SPP	suprapubic prostatectomy
SNT	suppan nail technique	SPROM	spontaneous premature rupture of membrane
S-O	salpingo-oophorectomy		
SOA	swelling of ankles; supraorbital artery	SPT	skin prick test
		SP TAP	spinal tap
SOAA	signed out against advice	SPU	short procedure unit
SOAP	subjective, objective, assessment and plan	SPV	systemic peripheral vascular resistance

SQ	subcutaneous
Sq CCa	squamous cell carcinoma
SR	sedimentation rate; sustained release; side rails; system review; sinus rhythm
SRBC	sickle/sheep red blood cells
SRBOW	spontaneous rupture of bag of waters
SRC	scleroderma renal crisis
Sr Cr	serum creatinine
SRF	somatotropin releasing factor
SRF-A	slow releasing factor of anaphylaxis
SRIF	somatotropin-release-inhibiting factor
SRMD	stress related mucosal dmage
SR/NE	sinus rhythm, no ectopy
SRNS	steroid responsive nephrotic syndrome
SROM	spontaneous rupture of membrane
SRS-A	slow reacting substance of anaphylaxis
SRT	speech reception threshold; sedimentation rate test
SRU	side rails up
SS	saline solution; salt substitute; sickle cell; social security/service; slip sent; symmetrical strength
S & S	signs and symptoms
SSCA	single shoulder contrast arthrography
SSD	social security disability; source to skin distance
SSDI	social security disability income
SSE	saline solution/soapsuds enema; systemic side effects
SSEPs	somatosensory evoked potentials
SSM	superficial spreading melanoma
SSOP	Second Surgical Opinion Program
SSPE	subacute sclerosing panencephalitis

SSS	sick sinus syndrome; sterile saline soak
SSSS	staphylococcal scalded skin syndrome
ST	speech therapist; sinus tachycardia; split thickness
STA	superficial temporal artery
stab	polymorphonuclear leukocytes in nonmature form
staph	Staphylococcus aureus
stat	immediately
STB	stillborn
ST BY	stand by
STD	sexually transmitted disease; skin test dose
STD TF	standard tube feeding
STET	submaximal treadmill exercise test
STF	special tube feeding
STG	short term goals
STH	soft tissue hemorrhage; somatotrophic hormone
STJ	subtalar joint
STM	short term memory
sTNM	surgical-evaluative staging of cancer
STNR	symmetrical tonic neck reflex
STORCH	syphilis, toxoplasmosis, other agents, rubella, cytomegalovirus and herpes
STPD	standard temperature and pressure-dry
strep	streptococcus
STS	serologic test for syphilis
STSG	split thickness skin graft
STU	shock trauma unit
S & U	supine and upright
SU	sensory urgency; Somogyi units
SUB	Skene's urethra and Bartholin's glands
sub q	subcutaneous
SUD	sudden unexpected death
SUID	sudden unexplained infant death
SUP	supinator; superior
supp	suppository
SUR	surgery; surgical

SV	single ventricle; stock volume; sigmoid volvulus	TAH	total abdominal hysterectomy; total artificial heart
SVC	superior vena cava	TAL	tendon Achilles lengthening
SVCO	superior vena cava obstruction	TANI	total axial node irradiation
SVD	spontaneous vaginal delivery	TAO	thromboangiitis obliterans
SVE	sterile vaginal examination	TAPVC	total anomalous pulmonary venous connection
SVPB	supraventricular premature beat		
		TAPVD	total anomalous pulmonary venous drainage
SVR	supraventricular rhythm; systemic vascular resistance		
		TAPVR	total anomalous pulmonary venous return
SVRI	systemic vascular resistance index		
		TAR	thrombocytopenia with absent radius
SVT	supraventricular tachycardia		
SW	social worker		
SWD	short wave diathermy	TARA	total articular replacement arthroplasty
SWFI	sterile water for injection		
SWI	sterile water for injection	TAS	therapeutics activities specialist
SWOG	Southwest Oncology Group		
SWS	slow wave sleep; Sturge-Weber syndrome; student ward secretary	TAT	tetanus antitoxin; till all taken; Thematic Apperception Test
		TB	tuberculosis
SWT	stab wound of the throat	TBA	to be admitted; to be absorbed
Sx	symptom; signs; surgery	TBB	transbronchial biopsy
SZ	seizure; suction; schizophrenic	tbc	tuberculosis
		TBE	tick-borne encephalitis
T	temperature	TBG	thyroxine-binding globulin
T$_{1/2}$	half-life	TBI	total body irradiation
T1	tricuspid first sound; first thoracic vertebra	T bili	total bilirubin
		tbl	tablespoon (15 mL)
T-7	free thyroxine factor	TBM	tubule basement membrane
TA	therapeutic abortion; temperature axillary; tricuspid atresia	TBNA	treated but not admitted
		TBPA	thyroxine-binding prealbumin
		TBR	total bed rest
Ta	tonometry applanation	TBSA	total burn surface area
T & A	tonsillectomy and adenoidectomy	tbsp	tablespoon (15 mL)
		TBV	total blood volume; transluminal balloon valvuloplasty
T(A)	axillary temperature		
TAA	total ankle arthroplasty; thoracic aortic aneurysm; tumor associated antigen (antibodies); transverse aortic arch		
		TBW	total body water
		T/C	to consider
		TC	throat culture; true conjugate
TAB	therapeutic abortion; triple antibiotic; tablet	T & C	type and crossmatch; turn and cough
TAD	transverse abdominal diameter	TCA	tricuspid atresia; terminal cancer
TAE	transcatheter arterial embolization		
		TCABG	triple coronary artery bypass graft
TAF	tissue angiogenesis factor		

TCBS agar	thiosulfate-citrate-bile salt-sucrose agar
TCCB	transitional cell carcinoma of bladder
TCDB	turn, cough and deep breathe
T cell	small lymphocyte
TCH	turn, cough, hyperventilate
TCID50	median tissue culture doses
TCM	transcutaneous monitor; tissue culture media
TCMH	tumor-direct cell-mediated hypersensitivity
TCVA	thromboembolic cerebral vascular accident
TD	tardive dyskinesia; travelers diarrhea; Takayasu's disease; transverse diameter; tidal volume; treatment discontinued; tetanus-diphtheria toxoid
Td	tetanus-diphtheria toxoid
TDD	thoracic duct drainage
TDE	total daily energy (requirement)
TDF	tumor dose fractionation
TDK	tardive dyskinesia
TDM	therapeutic drug monitoring
TdP	torsade de pointes
TDT	tentative discharge tomorrow
TE	tracheoesophageal; trace elements; thromboembolism
T & E	trial and error
TEA	total elbow arthroplasty; thromboendarterectomy
TEC	total eosinophil count
TEDS®	anti-embolism stockings
TEF	tracheoesophageal fistula
TEG	thromboelastogram
tele	telemetry
TEM	transmission electron microscopy
TEN	toxic epidermal necrolysis
TEN®	total enteral nutrition
TENS	transcutaneous electrical nerve stimulation
tert	tertiary
TES	trace element solution
TET	treadmill exercise test

TF	tetralogy of Fallot; tactile fremitus; tube feeding; to follow
TFB	trifascicular block
TFTs	thyroid function tests
TG	triglycerides
TGA	transient global amnesia; transposition of the great arteries
TGF	tissue/transforming growth factor
TGFA	triglyceride fatty acid
TGS	tincture of green soap
TGT	thromboplatin generation test
TH	total hysterectomy; thyroid hormone; thrill
THA	total hip arthroplasty; transient hemispheric attack
THC	transhepatic cholangiogram
TH-CULT	throat culture
THE	transhepatic embolization
Ther Ex	therapeutic exercise
THI	transient hypogammaglobinemia of infancy
THR	total hip replacement
TI	tricuspid insufficiency
tib	tibia
TIE	transient ischemia episode
TIG	tetanus immune globulin
TIN	tubulointerstitial nephritis
tinct	tincture
TJ	triceps jerk
TJN	twin jet nebulizer
TKA	total knee arthroplasty
TKNO	to keep needle open
TKP	thermokeratoplasty
TKO	to keep open
TKR	total knee replacement
TL	tubal ligation; team leader; trial leave
TLC	triple lumen catheter; thin layer chromatography; total lung capacity; total lymphocyte count; tender loving care
TLI	total lymphoid irradiation
TLS	tumor lysis syndrome
TLV	total lung volume

TM	tympanic membrane; trabecular meshwork	**TPM**	temporary pacemaker
TMA	transmetatarsal amputation	**TPN**	total parenteral nutrition
TMB	transient monocular blindness	**TP & P**	time, place and person
TMC	transmural colitis	**TPPE**	time, person, place and event
TMET	tread mill exercise test	**TPPN**	total peripheral parenteral nutrition
TMI	threatened myocardial infarction	**TPR**	temperature, pulse and respiration; temperature; total peripheral resistance
TMJ	temporomandibular joint		
TMP	trimethoprim; thallium myocardial perfusion	**TPT**	time to peak tension
		TPVR	total peripheral vascular resistance
TMS	trace metal solution		
TMTC	too many to count	**Tr**	trace; tremor; treatment; tincture
Tn	normal intraocular tension		
TNF	tumor necrosis factor	**T(R)**	rectal temperature
TNI	total nodal irradiation	**TRA**	therapeutic recreation associate
TNM	tumor node metastasis		
TNTC	too numerous to count	**trach**	tracheal; tracheostomy
TO	telephone order	**Trans D**	transverse diameter
T(O)	oral temperature	**TRC**	tanned red cells
TOA	tubo-ovarian abscess; time of arrival	**TRD**	traction retinal detachment
		Tren	Trendelenberg
TOF	tetralogy of Fallot	**TRH**	thyrotropin-releasing hormone
TOGV	transposition of the great vessels	**TRIG**	triglycerides
		tRNA	transfer ribonucleic acid
TOL	trial of labor	**TRNG**	tetracycline resistant Neisseria gonorrhea
tomo	tomography		
TOP	termination of pregnancy	**TRP**	tubular reabsorption of phosphate
TOPP	a drug combination protocol		
TOPV	trivalent oral polio vaccine	**TRT**	thermoradiotherapy
TORCH	toxoplasmosis, other (syphilis, hepatitis, Zoster), rubella, cytomegalovirus, and herpes simplex	**T3RU**	triiodothyroxine resin uptake
		TS	test solution; Tourette's syndrome
		TSA	total shoulder arthroplasty
TORP	total ossicular replacement prosthesis	**TSAR®**	tape surrounded Appli-rulers®
		TSBB	transtracheal selective bronchial brushing
TOS	thoracic outlet syndrome		
TP	total protein; Todd's paralysis	**TSD**	Tay-Sachs disease; target to skin distance
TPA	tissue plasminogen activator; tissue polypeptide antigen; total parenteral alimentation		
		T set	tracheotomy set
		TSF	tricep skin fold
TPC	total patient care	**TSH**	thyroid stimulating hormone
TPD	tropical pancreatic diabetes	**tsp**	teaspoon (5 mL)
TPE	total protective environment	**TSP**	total serum protein
TPH	thromboembolic pulmonary hypertension	**TSR**	total shoulder replacement
		TSS	toxic shock syndrome
TPI	Treponema pallidum immobilization test	**TST**	titmus stereocuity test
		T & T	touch and tone

TT	thrombin time; thymol turbidity; twitch tension; transtracheal; tilt table
TT_3	total serum triiodothyronine
TT_4	total thyroxine
TTA	total toe arthroplasty
TTN	transient tachypnea of the newborn
TTNB	transient tachypnea of the newborn
TTP	thrombotic thrombocytopenic purpura
TTS	through the skin
TTVP	temporary transvenous pacemaker
TU	tuberculin units
TUR	transurethral resection
T_3UR	triiodothyronine uptake ratio
TURB	turbidity
TURBN	transurethral resection bladder tumor
TURP	transurethral resection of prostate
TURV	transurethral resection valves
TV	tidal volume; trial visit; Trichomonas vaginalis
TVC	triple voiding cystogram; true vocal cord
TVH	total vaginal hysterectomy
TVP	transvenous pacemaker
TW	test weight
TWD	total white/differential count
TWE	tapwater enema
TWETC	tapwater enema till clear
TWWD	tap water wet dressing
Tx	treatment; therapy; traction; transfuse; transplant
TxA_2	thromboxane A_2
Tyl	tyloma
U	units; urine
U/1	1 finger breadth below umbilicus
1/U	1 finger over umbilicus
U/	at umbilicus
UA	uric acid; urinalysis; unauthorized absence; uncertain about
UAC	umbilical artery
UAE	urinary albumin excretion
UAL	umbilical artery line
UAO	upper airway obstruction
UAT	up as tolerated
UAVC	univentricular atrioventricular connection
UBF	unknown black female
UBI	ultraviolet blood irradiation
UBM	unknown black male
UC	urine culture; urethral catheter; uterine contraction; ulcerative colitis
U & C	urethral and cervical
UCD	usual childhood diseases
UCG	urinary chorionic-gonadotropins
UCHD	usual childhood diseases
UCI	urethral catheter in
UCO	urethral catheter out
UCX	urine culture
UD	urethral discharge
UDC	usual diseases of childhood
UE	upper extremity
UES	upper esophageal sphincter
UFO	unflagged order
UG	urogenital
UGDP	University Group Diabetes Project
UGH	uveitis, glaucoma, hyphema
UGI	upper gastrointestinal series
UHBI	upper hemibody irradiation
UHDDS	Uniform Hospital Discharge Data Set
UID	once daily
UIQ	upper inner quadrant
U/L	upper and lower
U & L	upper and lower
ULN	upper limits of normal
ULQ	upper left quadrant
UK	urokinase; unknown
UN	urinary nitrogen
UNA	urinary nitrogen appearance; urine sodium
ung	ointment
UNK	unknown
UOQ	upper outer quadrant
UPJ	ureteropelvic junction

U/P ratio	urine to plasma ratio	**VAS RAD**	vascular radiology
UPT	urine pregnancy test	**VB**	VanBuren (catheter)
UR	utilization review	**VBAC**	vaginal birth after cesarean
URI	upper respiratory infection	**VBI**	vertebrobasilar insufficiency
urol	urology	**VBS**	vertebral-basilar system
US	ultrasonography; unit secretary	**VC**	vital capacity; vena cava; vocal cords; color vision
USA	unit services assistant		
USB	upper sternal border	**VCG**	vectocardiography
USG	ultrasonography	**VCT**	venous clotting time
USI	urinary stress incontinence	**VCU**	voiding cystourethrogram
USN	ultrasonic nebulizer	**VCUG**	vesicoureterogram; voiding cystourethrogram
USP	United States Pharmacopeia		
USRDS	United States Renal Data System	**VD**	venereal disease; volume of distribution; voided
UTD	up to date	**VDA**	visual discriminatory acuity; venous digital angiogram
ut dict	as directed		
UTF	usual throat flora	**VDG**	venereal disease-gonorrhea
UTI	urinary tract infection	**VDH**	valvular disease of the heart
UTO	upper tibial osteotomy	**VDRL**	Venereal Disease Research Laboratory (test for syphilis)
UTZ	ultrasound		
UUN	urine urea nitrogen	**VDRR**	vitamin D-resistant rickets
UV	ultraviolet	**VDS**	venereal disease-syphilis
UVA	ultraviolet A light; ureterovesical angle	**VDT**	video display terminal
		VE	vaginal examination; vertex
UVB	ultraviolet B light	**VEB**	ventricular ectopic beat
UVC	umbilical vein catheter	**VEE**	Venezuelan equine encephalitis
UVJ	ureterovesical junction		
UVL	ultraviolet light	**vent**	ventricular; ventral
UWF	unknown white female	**VEP**	visual evoked potential
UWM	unknown white male	**VER**	visual evoked response; ventricular escape rhythm
V	vomiting; vein; vagina; five	**VF**	ventricular fibrillation; vision field; vocal fremitus
VA	Veterans Administration; visual acuity; vacuum aspiration		
		V fib	ventricular fibrillation
VAC	ventriculoarterial connections	**VFP**	vitreous fluorophotometry
VAD	vascular/venous access device	**VG**	vein graft; ventricular gallop; very good
vag	vagina		
VAG HYST	vaginal hysterectomy	**VH**	vaginal hysterectomy; viral hepatitis; vitreous hemorrhage; Veterans Hospital
VAH	Veterans Administration Hospital		
VAMC	Veterans Administraiton Medical Center		
		VI	volume index; six
VAPA	a drug combination protocol	**vib**	vibration
VAR	variant	**VID**	videodensitometry
VAS	vascular; visual analogue scale	**VIG**	vaccinia immune globulin
		VIP	voluntary interruption of pregnancy; vasoactive intestinal peptide
VASC	Visual-Auditory Screen Test for Children		

VISC	vitreous infusion suction cutter	VZIG	varicella zoster immune globulin
VIT	vitamin; vital; venom immunotherapy	VZV	varicella zoster virus
vit cap	vital capacity		
VKC	vernal keratoconjunctivitis	w	white; with; widowed
VLBW	very low birth weight	WA	while awake; when awake
VLDL	very low density lipoprotein	WAIS	Weschsler Adult Intelligence Scale
VLH	ventrolateral nucleus of the hypothalmus	WAIS-R	Wechsler Adult Intelligence Scale-Revised
VMH	ventromedial hypothalmus	WAP	wandering atrial pacemaker
VNA	Visiting Nurses Association	WAS	Wishott-Aldrich syndrome
VO	verbal order	WASS	Wasserman test
VOCTOR	void on call to operating room	WB	whole blood; weight bearing
VOD	vision right eye; venocclusive disease	WBAT	weight bearing as tolerated
VOL	voluntary	WBC	white blood cell/count
VOR	vestibular ocular reflex	WBH	whole-body hyperthermia
VOS	vision left eye	WBN	wellborn nursery
VOU	vision both eyes	WC	wheelchair; white count; ward clerk; whooping cough
VP	venous pressure; variegate porphyria; ventriculoperitoneal; ventricular-peritoneal	W/D	warm and dry; withdrawal
		W-D	wet to dry
V & P	ventilation and perfusion; vagotomy and pyloroplasty	WDHA	watery diarrhea, hypokalemia and achlorhydria
VPB	ventricular premature beat	WDL	well-differentiated lymphocyte
VPC	ventricular premature contractions	WDLL	well-differentiated lymphocytic lymphoma
VPDs	ventricular premature depolarizations	WDWN-BF	well-developed, well-nourished black female
VPL	vento-posterolateral	WDWN-BM	well-developed, well-nourished black male
VR	ventricular rhythm; verbal reprimand	WDWN-WF	well-developed, well nourished white female
VS	vital signs; versus	WDWN-WM	well-developed, well-nourished white male
VSD	venous stasis retinopathy		
VSS	vital signs stable	WE	weekend
VT	ventricular tachycardia	WEE	western equine encephalitis
v tach	ventricular tachycardia	WEP	weekend pass
VTE	venous thromboembolism	WF	white female
VTX	vertex	WFI	water for injection
VV	varicose veins	WFL	within functional limits
V & V	vulva and vagina	WFR	wheel-and-flare reaction
V/V	volume to volume ratio	WHO	World Health Organization
VVFR	vesicovaginal fistula repair	WHV	woodchuck hepatitis virus
VVOR	visual-vestibulo-ocular-reflex	WHVP	wedged hepatic venous pressure
VW	vessel wall	WIA	wounded in action
VWM	ventricular wall motion	WIC	women, infants and children
VZ	varicella zoster		

WID	widow; widower	**XM**	crossmatch
WISC	Welcher Intelligence Scale for Children	**X-mat**	crossmatch
		XMM	xeromammography
WLS	wet lung syndrome	**XRT**	radiotherapy
WLT	waterload test	**XS-LIM**	exceeds limits of procedure
WKS	Wernicke-Korsakoff syndrome	**XT**	exotropia
WM	white male	**XX**	normal female sex chromosome type
WMA	wall motion abnormality		
WN	well nourished	**XY**	normal male sex chromosome type
WND	wound		
WNL	within normal limits		
W/O	without	**YACP**	young adult chronic patient
WO	written order; weeks old	**YAG**	yittrium aluminum garnert (laser)
WP	whirlpool		
WPFM	Wright peak flow meter	**YF**	yellow fever
WPP	Welcher Preschool Primary Scale of Intelligence	**YJV**	yellow jacket venom
		YLC	youngest living child
WPW	Wolff-Parkinson-White	**YO**	years old
WR	Wasserman reaction; wrist	**YORA**	younger-onset rheumatoid arthritis
WS	ward secretary; watt seconds		
wt	weight	**YSC**	yolk sac carcinoma
WWAC	walk with aid of cane		
W/U	workup	**ZEEP**	zero end-expiratory pressure
W/V	weight-to-volume ratio	**ZES**	Zollinger-Ellison syndrome
W/W	weight-to-weight ratio	**Z-ESR**	zeta erythrocyte sedimentation rate
X	crossmatch; start of anesthesia; except; times; ten; break	**ZIG**	zoster serum immune globulin
		ZIP	zoster immune plasma
X3	orientation as to person, place and time	**ZIZ**	zoster serum immune globulin
		ZMC	zygomatic
X & D	examination and diagnosis	**Zn**	zinc

DRUG/CHEMICAL ABBREVIATIONS

AA	amino acid
ABCDE	botulism toxoid pentavalent
ABDIC	(a drug combination protocol)
ABDV	(a drug combination protocol)
ABE	botulism equine trivalent antitoxin
ABVD	adriamycina, bleomycin, vinblastine and dacarbazine (DTIC)
5-AC	azacitidine
ACA	acyclovir
ACD	acid-citrate-dextroseanemia of chronic disease; dactinomycin
ACH	adrenal cortical hormone
ACh	acetylcholine
ACP	acid phosphatase
ACT-D	dactinomycin
ACTH	corticotropin (adrenocorticotrophic hormone)
ACV	acyclovir
ADA	adenosine deaminase
ADH	antidiuretic hormone
ADM	doxorubicin
Ad-OAP	doxorubicin/vincristine/ cytarabine/prednisone
ADP	adenosine diphosphate
ADR	doxorubicin (Adriamycin®)
AG	aminoglycoside
AgNO3	silver nitrate
AH	antihyaluronidase
AHA	acetohydroxamic acid
ALA	aminolevulinic acid
ALD	aldolase
Al(OH)3	aluminum hydroxide
AMP	adenosine monophosphate
m-AMSA	acridinyl anisidide
ANA	antinuclear antibody
ANF	atrial natriuretic factor
APAP	acetaminophen
APC	aspirin, phenacetin and caffeine
APO	(a drug combination protocol)
apo E	apolipoprotein E

APPG	aqueous procaine penicillin G
ARA-A	vidarabine
ARA-C	cytarabine
ASA	acetylsalicylic acid; argininosuccinate
ASK	antistreptokinase
ASL	antistreptolysin (titer)
ASLO	antistreptolysin-O
ASO	antistreptolysin-O
ASOT	antistreptolysin-O titer
ATP	adenosine triphosphate
ATPase	adenosine triphosphatase
AT 10	dihydrotachysterol
Au	gold
AVP	arginine vasopressin
AZA	azathioprine
5-AZA	azacitidine
AZQ	diaziquone
AZT	azidothymidine
B$_1$	thiamine HCl
B$_2$	riboflavin
B$_6$	pyridoxine HCl
B$_7$	biotin
B$_8$	adenosine phosphate
B$_{12}$	cyanocobalamin
Ba	barium
BAC	benzalkonium chloride
BACOP	bleomycin, adriamycin, cyclophosphamide, vincristine, prednisone
BAL	British antilewisite (dimercaprol)
BCNU	carmustine
BDP	beclomethasone diprorionate
BHC	benzene hexachloride
BHI	biosynthetic human insulin
BLEO	bleomycin sulfate
BLM	bleomycin sulfate
B & O	belladonna & opium
BOLD	bleomycin, vincristine (Oncovin®), lomustine, dacarbazine
BP	benzoyl peroxide
BPL	benzylpenicilloyl-polylysine

BPN	bacitracin, polymyxin B, neomycin sulfate
BSF	busulfan
BSP	bromsulfophalein
BSSG	sitogluside
BUdR	bromodeoxyurdine
BZ	phenylbutazone
BZDZ	benzodiazepine
CACP	cisplatin
CAF	cyclophosphamide, doxorubicin, fluorouracil
CAMF	cyclophosphamide, adriamycin, methotrexate, fluorouracil
CAMP	cyclophosphamide, doxorubicin, methotrexate, procarbazine
CAP	cyclophosphamide, doxorubicin, cisplatin
CAV	cyclophosphamide, doxorubicin, vincristine
CBC	carbenicillin
CBD	cannabidial
CBZ	carbamazepine
CCB	calcium channel blocker
CCFE	cyclophosphamide, cisplatin, fluorouracil, estramustine
CCK	cholecystokinin
CCK-OP	cholecystokinin octapeptide
CCK-PZ	cholecystokinn-pancreozymin
CCM	cyclophosphamide, lomustine, methotrexate
CCNU	lomustine
CCT in PET	crude coal tar in petroleum
CDA	chenodeoxycholic acid (chenodiol)
CDC	chenodeoxycholic acid
CDCA	chenodeoxycholic acid (chenodiol)
CDDP	cisplatin
CEPH	cephalosporin
CF	calcium leucovorin; cephalothin
CHAD	cyclophosphamide, adriamycin, cisplatin, hexamethylmelamine
CH3-CCNU	semustine

CHOP	cyclophosphamide, doxorubicin, vincristine, prednisone
CISCA	cisplatin, Cytoxan®, Adriamycin®
CLB	chlorambucil
CLO	cod liver oil
CM	capreomycin
CMC	chloramphenicol; carboxymethylcellulose
CMF	cyclophosphamide, methotrexate, fluorouracil
CMFVP	cyclophosphamide, methotrexate, fluorouracil, vincristine, prednisone
CMOPP	a drug combination protocol
CMP	chloramphenicol
CNCbl	cyanocobalamin
CNF	cyclophosphamide, mitoxantrone, fluorouracil
CO	castor oil
COAP	cyclophosphamide, vincristine, cytarabine, prednisone
COD	codeine
COHB	carboxyhemoglobin
Coke	cocaine
COMLA	a drug combination protocol
CON A	concanavalin A
CONPA-DRI I	cyclophosphamide, vincristine, doxorubicin, melphalan
CONPA-DRI II	conpadri I plus high dose methotrexate
CONPA-DRI 3	conpadri I plus intensified doxorubicin
COP	cyclophosphamide, vincristine, prednisone
COP-BLAM	a drug combination protocol
COPP	cyclophosphamide, vincristine, procarbazine, prednisone
CPD	citrate-phosphate-dextrose
CPM	cyclophosphamide; chlorpheniramine maleate; chlorpropamide
CPPD	cisplatin; calcium pyrophosphate dihydrate
CPZ	chlorpromazine; Compazine®
CS	cycloserine
CsA	cyclosporin

CSB	caffeine sodium benzoate		DHAD	mitoxanthrone HCl
CSP	cellulose sodium phosphate		DHE 45®	dihydroergotamine mesylate
CT	calcitonin		DHEA	dehydroepiandrosterone
CTM	Chlor-Trimeton®		DHT	dihydrotachysterol
CTX	cyclophosphamide (Cytoxan®)		DIC	dacarbazine
CVP	a drug combination protocol		dig	digoxin; digitoxin (Note: confusing)
CyA	cyclosporine			
CYT	cyclophosphamide		D5LR	dextrose 5% in lactated Ringer's injection
Cyclo C	cyclocytidine HCl			
CY-VA-DIC	cyclophosphamide, vincristine, adriamycin, dacarbazine		DM	dextromethorphan
			DMBA	dimethylbenzatracene
CZI	crystalline zinc insulin		DMI	desipramine
CZN	chlorzotocin		DMO	dimethadone
D	cholecalciferol		DMSO	dimethyl sulfoxide
DA	dopamine		DMT	dimethyltryptamine
DACT	dactinomycin		DNA	deoxyribonucleic acid
DAG	dianhydrogalactitol		DNCB	dinitrochlorobenzene
DAM	diacetylmonoxine		D5NS	5% dextrose in normal saline
DAT	daunorubicin, cytaribine (ARA-C), thioguanine		D5NSS	5% dextrose in normal saline solution
DBD	milolactol (dibromodulicitol)		DOB	dobutamine
DBED	penicillin G benzathine		DOCA	desoxycorticosterone acetate
DBI®	phenformin HCl		DOP	dopamine
DBQ	debrisoquin		DOSS	docusate sodium (dioctyl sodium sulfosuccinate)
DBZ	dibenzamine			
DC65®	Darvon Compound 65®		2,3-DPG	2,3-diphosphoglyceric acid
DCMXT	dichloromethotrexate		DPH	phenytoin; diphenhydramine
DCN	Darvocet-N®		DPT	Demerol®, Phenergan® & Thorazine®
DCNU	chlorozotocin			
DCP®	calcium phosphate, dibasic		D/S	5% dextrose and 0.9% sodium chloride injection
DDAVP®	desmopressin acetate			
DDP	cisplatin		D5S	dextrose 5% in saline
DDS	dapsone		DSI	deep shock insulin
DDT	chlorophenothane; dichloro-diphenyl-trichlorome thylmethane		DSS	docusate sodium
			DT	diptheria tetanus/toxoid
			DTBC	d-tubocurarine (tubocurarine)
DEC	diethylcarbamazine		DTIC	dacarbazine
Deet	diethyltoluamide		DTPA	pentetic acid (diethylenetriamine-penta-acetic acid)
DES	diethylstilbestrol			
DET	diethyltryptamine			
DFD	diisopropyl phosphorofluoridate		DTT	diphtheria tetanus toxoid
			DVA	vindesine
DFO	deferoxamine		D5W	5% dextrose in water injection
DFOM	deferoxamine		DW	dextrose in water; distilled water; deionized water
DFP	diisopropyl flurophosphate (isoflurophane)			
			DXM	dexamethasone
DHA	docosahexaenoic acid; dihydroxyacetone		EACA	aminocaproic acid
			ECA	ethacrynic acid

ECHO	etoposide, cyclophosphamide, Adriamycin®, vincristine
EDTA	ethylene-dinitrilo tetraacetic acid (edetic acid)
EES®	erythromycin ethylsuccinate
EHDA	etidronate sodium
EMB	ethambutol
EOG	Ethrane®, oxygen and gas
EPA	eicosapentaenoic acid
EPEG	etoposide
EPI	epinephrine
ETA	ethionamide
ETH	elixir terpin hydrate; ethanol
ETH&C	elixir terpin hydrate with codeine
EtO	ethylene oxide
ETOH	alcohol
FAC	fluorouracil, Adriamycin®, cyclophosphamide
FAM	fluorouracil, Adriamycin®, mitomycin
FBH	hydroxybutyric dehydrogenase
5-FC	flucytosine
FeSO$_4$	ferrous sulfate
FIGLU	formininoglutamic acid
FITC	fluorescein isothiocynate
FML®	fluorometholone
FOG	Fluothane®, oxygen and gas (nitrous oxide)
FOMI	fluorouracil, Oncovin® (vincristine), and mitomycin
FPZ	fluphenazine
FPZ-D	fluphenazine decanoate
FT$_3$	free triiodothyroxine
FT$_4$	free thyroxine
F$_3$T	trifluridine
5-FU	fluorouracil
FUDR®	floxuridine
G-11	hexachlorophene
GABA	gamma-aminobutyric acid
GAG	glycosaminoglycan
GBH	gamma benzene hexachloride (lindane)
GENT	gentamicin
GG	gamma globulin; guaifenesin (glyceryl guaicolate)
GHB	gamma hydroxybutyrate
GIK	glucose-insulin-potassium
GMP	guanosine monophosphate
GOT	glutamic-oxaloacetic transaminase; aspartate aminotransferase
G6PD	glucose-6-phosphate dehydrogenase
GPT	glutamic pyruvic transaminase
GST	gold sodium thiomalate
GTP	glutamyl transpeptidase
HBD	hydroxybutyric acid dehydrogenase
HC	hydrocortisone
HCl	hydrochloric acid; hydrochloride
HCO$_3$	bicarbonate
HCTZ	hydrochlorothiazide
HDARAC	high dose cytarabine
HDMTX	high-dose methotrexate
H & E	hematoxylin and eosin
Hex	hexamethylmelamine
HGPRT	hypoxanthine-guanine phosphoribosyltransferase
5-HIAA	5 hydroxyindolacetic acid
HIDA	hepato-iminodiacetic acid
HL	haloperidol
HL-D	haloperidol decanoate
HM	human semisynthetic insulin
HMB	homatropine methylbromide
HMG CoA	hepatic hydroxymethylglutaryl coenzyme A
HMM	hexamethylmelamine
HMP	hexose monophosphate
HN$_2$	mechlorethamine HCl
HNRNA	heterogeneous nuclear ribonucleic acid
H$_2$O	water
H$_2$O$_2$	hydrogen peroxide
HP	hydrophilic petrolatum
HPO	hhydrophilic ointment
HQC	hydroquinone cream
HSA	human serum albumin
5-HT	5-hydroxytryptamine
5-HTP	5-hydroxytryptophan
HUR	hydroxyurea
HXM	hexamethylmelamine
ICD	isocitrate dehydrogenase
ICRF-159	razoxane
IDU	idoxuridine

IF	interferon	Mg	magnesium
IFN	interferon	MgO	magnesium oxide
IL	Intralipid®; interleukin	MgSO$_4$	magnesium sulfate
IMI	iimipramine	MHB	methemoglobin
INH	isoniazid	MIF	merthiolate-iodine-formalin
IPA	isopropyl alcohol	MISO	misonidazole
ISDN	isosorbide dinitrate	MITO-C	mitomycin
ISO	isoproterenol	M & M	Maalone® and merthiolate
IVA	Intervir-A	MMC	mitomycin C
K	potassium; vitamin K	Mn	manganese
K$_1$	phytonadione	MO	mineral oil
K$_3$	menadione	Mo	molybdenum
K$_4$	menadiol sodium diphosphate	MOF	methotrexate, Oncovin®, and fluorouracil
KCl	potassium chloride		
KI	potassium iodide	MOM	milk of magnesia
KM	kanamycin	MOPP	mechlorethamine, vincristine, procarbazine, prednisone
KMnO$_4$	potassium permanganate		
KOH	potassium hydroxide	MP	mercaptopurine
L	lente insulin	6-MP	mercaptopurine
LAS	leucine acetylsalicylate	MPH	methylphenidate
L-ASP	asparaginase	MS	morphine sulfate
LCAT	lecithin cholesterol acyltransferase	MSG	monosodium glutamate; methysergide
LCD	liquor carbonis detergens (coal tar solution)	MSH	melanocyte-stimulating hormone
LD	levodopa; lactic dehydrogenase	MSO$_4$	morphine sulfate
		MTU	methylthiouracil
LI	lithium	MTX	methotrexate
LICO$_3$	lithium carbonate	Na	sodium
L-PAM	melphalan	NaCl	sodium chloride
LR	lactated Ringer's (solution)	NADPH	nicotinamide adenine dinucleotide phosphate
LSD	lysergide; lysergic acid diethylamide		
		NaF	sodium fluoride
L-Spar	Elspar® (asparaginase)	NaHCO$_3$	sodium bicarbonate
mag cit	magnesium citrate	NaI	sodium iodide
mag sulf	magnesium sulfate	NAPA	N-acetyl procainamide
MAOI	monoamine oxidase inhibitor	Na Pent	Pentothal Sodium®
M-BACOD	a drug combination protocol	NCAS	neocarzinostatin
MC	monocomponent highly purified pork insulin	NCS	zinostatis (neocarzinostatin)
		Nd	neodymium
MDA	methylenedioxyamphetamine	NE	norepinephrine
MDP	methylene diphosphorate	NH$_4$Cl	ammonium chloride
MeCCNU	semustine	nitro	nitroglycerin
METH b	methemoglobin	N$_2$O	nitrous oxide
MEL B	melarsoprol	N$_2$O:O$_2$	nitrous oxide to oxygen ratio
MGBG	methyl-GAG (methylglyoxal bisguanylhydrazone)	NOR	nortriptyline
		NOR-EPI	norepinephrine
		NP	neurophysin

NPH	neutral protamine Haedorn insulin
NS	normal saline
NSAIA	non-steroidal anti-inflammatory agent
NSAID	non-steroidal anti-inflammatory drug
NSO	Neosporin® ointment
NSS	sodium chloride 0.9%; normal saline solution
1/2 NSS	sodium chloride 0.45%
NTG	nitroglycerin
NTP	Nitropaste®; sodium nitroprusside
NZ	enzyme
OCT	ornithine carbamyl transferase
17 OH	17-hydroxycorticosteroids
OHA	oral hypoglycemic agents
OH Cbl	hydroxycobalamine
OHD	hydroxy vitamin D
OHG	oral hypoglycemic
OHIAA	hydroxyindolacetic acid
ON	Ortho-Novum®
OS	osmium
32P	radioactive phosphorus
PA	phenol alcohol
PAH	para-aminohippurate
PAM	penicillin aluminum monostearate
PAS/PASA	para-aminosalicyclic acid
Pb	phenobarbital
P & B	phenobarbital and belladonna
PBG	porphobilinogen
PBI	protein-bound iodine
PBN	polymyxin B sulfate, bacitracin and neomycin
PBZ	pyribenzamine; phenylbutazone; phenoxybenzamine
PCB	pancuronium bromide; polychlorinated biphenyl
PCMX	chloroxylenol
PCN	penicillin
PCP	phencyclidine; polychlorinated biphenyl
PCZ	prochlorperazine; procarbazine
PDD	cisplatin

PDN	prednisone
PE	polyethylene
P_1E_1®	epinephrine 1%, pilocarpine 1% ophthalmic solution
PEG	polyethylene glycol
PETN	pentaerythritol tetranitrate
PG	paregoric; polygalacturonate; phosphatidyl glycerol
PGA	prostaglandin
PGE2	prostaglandin E2
PHT	phenytoin
PIO	pemoline
Pit	Pitocin®; Pitressin®
PO_4	phosphate
POMP	prednisone, vincristine, methotrexate, mercaptopurine
PPA	phenylpropanolamine
PPD	purified protein derivative (of tuberculin)
Pred	prednisone
PRL	prolactin
PRM-SDX	pyrimethamine sulfadoxine
ProMACE	a drug protocol combination
PRP	polyribose ribitol phosphate; panretinal photocoagulation
PRPP	5-phosphoribosyl-1-pyrophosphate
PRZF	pyrazofurin
PSP	phenolsulphthalein
PT	phenytoin
PTA	phosphotungstic acid
PTC	phenylthiocarbamoxl
PTFE	polytetrafluorethylene
PTG	teniposide
PTL	Sodium Pentothal®
PTU	propylthiouracil
PVA	polyvinyl alcohol
PVC	polyvinyl chloride
PVK	penicillin V potassium
PVP	polyvinyl-pyrrolidone
PZA	pyrazinamide
PZI	protamine zinc insulin
RAA	renin-angiotensin-aldosterone
RAI	radioactive iodine
RI	regular insulin
RIF	rifampin
RIG	rabies immune globulin

RMS®	Rectal Morphine Sulfate		**TBX$_2$**	thromboxane B$_2$
RNA	ribonucleic acid		**TBX®**	thiabendazole
rRNA	ribosomal ribonucleic acid		**TC**	transcobalamin; tubocurarine
RS	Ringer's solution		**Tc**	technetium
S	semilente insulin		**TCA**	tricyclic antidepressant;
SA	salicylic acid			trichloroacetic acid
SAS	sulfasalazine		**TCAD**	tricyclic antidepressant
SBC	standard bicarbonate		**TCBS**	thiosulfate-citrate-bile
SCG	sodium cromoglycate			salt-sucrose agar
SCh	succinylcholine chloride		**TCDD**	tetrachlorodibenzop-dioxin
SCOP	scopolamine		**TCE**	tetrachloroethylene
SCP	sodium cellulose phosphate		**TCMZ**	trichloromethiazide
SK	streptokinase		**TCN**	tetracycline
SK 65®	propoxyphene HCl 65 mg		**TCT**	thyrocalcitonin
SK-SD	streptokinase streptodornase		**TD**	tetanus-diphtheria toxoid
SLO	streptolysin O		**Td**	tetanus-diphtheria toxoid
SM	streptomycin		**TDI**	toluene diisocyanate
SMX-TMP	sulfamethoxazole/trimethoprim		**TdR**	thymidine
SMZ-TMP	sulfamethoxazole/trimethoprim		**TESPA**	thiotepa
SNP	sodium nitroprusside		**TFT**	trifluridine (trifluorothymidine)
SO$_4$	sulfate		**6-TG**	thioguanine
SOD	superoxide dysmutase		**TGFA**	triglyceride fatty acid
SPS	sodium polyethanol sulfanate		**TGS**	tincture of green soap
SRT	sustained release theophylline		**THAM®**	tromethamine
SS	saline solution		**THC**	tetrahydrocannibinol
SSD	silver sulfadiazine		**THP**	trihexphenidyl
SSI	sub-shock insulin		**TMC**	triamcinolone; Terramycin®
SSKI	saturated solution potassium			capsules
	iodide		**TMP**	trimethoprim
SSX	sulfisoxazole acetyl		**TMP/SMX**	trimethoprim/sulfamethoxazole
STD	sodium tetradecyl sulfate		**TMP/SMZ**	trimethoprim/sulfamethoxazole
STP	sodium thiopental		**TMX**	tamoxifen
strep	streptomycin		**TNG**	nitroglycerin
STZ	streptozocin		**TOPV**	trivalent oral polio vaccine
SULF-PRIM	trimethoprim and		**TRH**	thyrotropin-releasing hormone
	sulfamethoxazole		**TRM-SMX**	trimethoprim-sulfamethoxazole
SUX	succinylcholine		**tRNA**	transfer ribonucleic acid
SZN	streptozocin		**TSA**	toluenesulfonic acid
T3	Tyleonol® #3		**TSH**	thyroid stimulating hormone
T$_3$	triiodothyronine		**TSPA**	thiotepa
T$_4$	levothyroxine		**TT**	tetanus toxoid
TAA	triamcinolone acetonide		**TT$_3$**	total serum triiodothyronine
TAB	triple antibiotic		**TT$_4$**	total thyroxine
TAC	triamicinolone cream		**TxA$_2$**	thromboxane A$_2$
TAM	tamoxifen		**Tyl**	Tylenol®
TAO	troleandomycin		**TYCO #3**	Tylenol® with 30 mg of
TBG	thyroxine-binding globulin			codeine
TBPA	thyroxine-binding prealbumin		**U**	ultralente insulin

297

UK	urokinase	**VDS**	vindesine
VA	valproic acid	**VM 26**	teniposide
VAC	vincristine, Adriamycin®, cyclophosphamide	**VMA**	vanillymandelic acid
		VP-16	etoposide
VAPA	a drug combination protocol	**VPA**	valproic acid
VBD	vinblastine, bleomycin and cisplatin	**ZnO**	zinc oxide
		ZnOE	zinc oxide and eugenol
VBL	vinblastine	**ZPC**	zopiclone
VCR	vincristine sulfate		

298

TERMS USED IN PRESCRIPTION WRITING

TERM	MEANING	ABBREVIATION
acidum	an acid	acid, ac.
ad	to, up to	ad
adde, addatur	add, let be added	add.
ad libitum	as much as desired	ad lib.
admove, admoveatur	apply, let be applied	admov.
ad partes dolentes	to the painful parts	ad part. dolent.
agita, agitetur	shake, stir	agit.
albus, -a, -um	white	alb.
aluminum	aluminum	al.
ampulla	an ampul	ampul.
ana	of each	aa
ante	before	a.
ante cibos	before meals	a.c., ac
ante cibum	before food	a.c., ac
aqua	water	aq.
aqua bulliens	boiling water	aq. bull.
aqua destillata	distilled water	aq. dest.
balneum	bath	baln.
balneum vaporis	steam bath	baln. vap., b.v.
bene	well	bene
bis in die	twice a day	b.i.d., BID
bromidum	a bromide	brom.

calcium	calcium	*calc., Ca*
capsula, capsulae	capsule, capsules	*cap., caps.*
carbons	carbonate	*carb.*
cataplasma	a cataplasm, poultice	*catapl.*
charta, chartae	paper(s), powder(s)	*chart.*
charta cerata	waxed paper	*chart. cerat.*
chartula	(small) paper, powder	*chart.*
chloridum	chloride	*chlorid.*
cochleare amplum	tablespoonful	*coch. ampl\.*
cochleare magnum	tablespoonful	*coch. mag.*
cochleare parvum	teaspoonful	*coch. parv.*
collodium	collodion	*collod.*
collunarium	nasal douche	*collun.*
collyrium	eye lotion, eyewash	*collyr.*
compositus, -a, -um	compound	*comp., co.*
congius	gallon	*cong., C.*
cum	with	*c*
cum aqua	with water	*cum aq.*
cum cibos	with meals, food	*cc*
da, detur, dentur	give, let be given	*d., det.*
dentur tales doses	give of such doses	*d.t.d.DTD*
diebus alternis	on alternate days	*dieb. alt., QOD*
dilutus, -a, -um	dilute	*dil.*
dimidius, -a, -um	one half	*dim.*
dividatur in partes aequales	let be divided into equal parts	*div. in par. aeq.*
dosis	dose	*dos.*

durante dolare	while pain lasts	dur. dol.
elixir	an elixir	elix., el.
emplastrum	a plaster	emp.
emulsum	emulsion	emuls.
et	and	et
ex aqua	in water	ex aq.
ex modo praescripto	in the manner prescribed	e.m.p.
extractum	an extract	ext.
fac, fiat, fiant	make	ft.
ferrum	iron	ferr.
fiant	let them be made	ft.
fiat	let it be made	ft.
fiat lege artis	let be made according to the law of the art	f.l.a.
filtra	filter	filt.
gargarisma	a gargle	garg.
gelatum	a gel, jelly	gel.
glyceritum	a glycerite	glycer.
glycerogelatinum	glycerogelatin	glycerogel.
granum, grana	a grain, grains	gr.
gutta, guttae	drop, drops	gt., gtt.
guttatim	drop by drop	guttat.
hora decubitus	at bed hour, at bedtime	hor. decub., h.d.
hora somni	before sleep	h.s., HS
hydrargyrum	mercury	hydrarg.
in	in, into, within	in
in aqua	in water	in aq.

in die	in a day	_in d._
infusum	an infusion	_inf._
inhalatio	inhalation	_inhal._
in vitro	in glass	_in vit._
iodidum	an iodide	_iodid._
kalium	potassium	_K_
lavatio	a wash	_lavat._
leviter	lightly	_lev., levit._
linimentum	a linament	_lin._
liquor	a liquor, solution	_liq._
lotio	a lotion	_lot._
magma	a magma, milk	_mag._
magnesium	magnesium	_Mg_
magnus, -a, -um	large	_mag._
mane primo	first thing in the morning	_man. prim._
misce	you mix	_M._
mistura	a mixture	_mist._
mitte tales	send such	_mitt. tal._
modo dictu	as directed	_m. dict._
modo praescripto	in the manner prescribed	_mod. praes., m.p._
mollis	soft	_moll._
moro dicto	in the manner directed	_mor. dict._
mucilago	a mucilage	_mucil._
natrium	sodium	_Na_
nebula	a spray	_nebul._
nihil album	zinc oxide	_nihil alb._

nocte	at night	*noct.*
nocte maneque	night and morning	*noct. maneq.*
non repetatur	do not repeat	*non rep.*
octarius	a pint	*O., oct.*
oculo dextro	in the right eye	*ocul. dext., o.d., O.D.*
oculo sinistro	in the left eye	*ocul. sinist., o.s., O.S.*
oculo utro	each eye	*ocul. utro, o.u., O.U.*
odontalgicum	toothache drops	*odont.*
oleum	an oil	*ol.*
omni hora	every hour	*omn. hor., qh*
omni mane vel nocte	every morning or night	*omn. man. vel noct.*
omni quarta hora	every four hours	*omn. 4 hr., q4h*
omnis	all, every	*omn.*
omni secunda hora	every two hours	*omn. 2 hr, q2h*
omni tertia hora	every three hours	*omn. tert. hor., q3h*
optimus, -a, -um	the best	*opt.*
partes aequales	equal parts	*p.e., part. aeq.*
parvus, -a, -um	small	*parv.*
pasta	a paste	*pat.*
pastillus	lozenge, pastille	*pastil.*
per diem	per day	*per diem*
per os	by mouth	*per os, PO*
phosphas	a phosphatate	*phos.*
pilula, pilulae	a pill, pills	*pil.*
placebo	I please	*placebo*
ponderosus	heavy	*pond.*

post cibum, post cibos	after food, after meals	*p.c., PC*
praecipitatus	precipitated	*ppt.*
pro dose	for a dose	*pro dos.*
pro ratione aetatis	according to age	*pro rat. aet.*
pro recto	rectally	*pro rect.*
pro re nata	as occasion arises	*p.r.n., PRN*
pro urethra	urethral	*pro ureth*
pro usu externo	for external use	*pro us. ext.*
pro vagina	vaginal	*pro vagin.*
pulvis, pulveres	a powder, powders	*pulv.*
quantum libet/placet/vis	as much as you wish	*q.l., q.p., q.v.*
quantum sufficit	as much as suffices	*q.s., QS*
quaque die	every day	*q.d., QD*
quaque hora	every hour	*qq. hor., qh*
quater in die	four times a day	*q.i.d.*
recipe	take thou	*Rx.*
ruber, rubra, rubrum	red	*rub.*
sal	salt	*sal*
saturatus, -a, -um	saturated	*sat.*
secundum artem	according to art	*s.a.*
semel	once	*semel*
semi, semis	one half	*ss, sem.*
semihora	half hour	*semih.*
sesqui	one and one half	*sesq.*
signa, signetur	write, let it be written	*sig., S.*
simul	at the same time	*sumul*

sine	without	*s., w/o*
sine aqua	without water	*sine aq.*
si opus sit	if there is need	*si op. sit, s.o.s.*
sodium	sodium	*sod., Na*
solutio	a solution	*sol.*
solutio saturata	a saturated solution	*sol. sat.*
spiritus	a spirit	*sp.*
spiritus vini rectificatus	alcohol	*sp. vin. rect., s.v.r.*
spiritus vini tenuis	proof spirit, diluted alcohol	*sp. vin. ten., s.v.t.*
statim	immediately	*stat., STAT*
sume, sumendus	take, to be taken	*sum.*
suppositoria	suppositories	*suppos.*
suppositoria rectalia	rectal suppositories	*suppos. rect., RS*
suppositorium	a suppository	*suppos.*
syrupus	a syrup	*syr.*
tabletta	tablet	*tab.*
tales doses	such doses	*tal. dos.*
talis, tales, talia	such	*tal.*
ter	three times, thrice	*t.*
ter in die	three times a day	*t.i.d., TID*
tinctura	a tincture	*tr., tinct.*
trituratio	a trituration	*trit.*
trochiscus, trochisci	a troche, troches	*troch.*
uncia	ounce	*oz.*
unguentum	an ointment	*ungt.*
ut dictum	as told, as directed	*ut dict.*

vaccinum	a vaccine	*vac.*
vel	vel	*or*
vinum	a wine	*vin.*
viridis	green	*vir.*

TABLES OF
WEIGHTS AND MEASURES

THE METRIC SYSTEM

nano   —used to denote one billionth (10^{-9}) of the basic unit
micro   —used to denote one millionth of the basic unit
milli   —used to denote one thousandth of the basic unit
centi   —used to denote one hundredth of the basic unit
deci   —used to denote one tenth of the basic unit
deka   —used to denote ten times the basic unit
hekto   —used to denote one hundred times the basic unit
kilo   —used to denote one thousand times the basic unit

Table of Metric Weights

1 kilogram (kg)	= 1000 grams
1 gram (g)	= 1000 milligrams
1 milligram (mg)	= 0.001 gram
1 microgram (μg or mcg)	= 0.001 milligram
1 nanogram (ng)	= 0.001 microgram

Table of Metric Volumes

1 kiloliter (kl)	= 1000 liters
1 liter (L, l)	= 1000 ml
1 milliliter (ml)	= 0.001 liter
1 milliliter (ml)	= 0.001 liter
1 microliter (μl)	= 0.001 milliliter

Table of Metric Lengths

1 kilometer (km)	= 1000 meters
1 meter (M, m)	= 1000 millimeters
1 decimeter (dm)	= 100 millimeters
1 centimeter (cm)	= 10 millimeters
1 millimeter (mm)	= 0.001 meter
1 micrometer (μm)	= 0.001 millimeter
1 nanometer (nm)	= 0.000,000,001 meter

Apothecary Measures

Fluid Measure

60 minims (m)	= 1 fluidrachm (fl dr)
8 fluidrachms (480 minims)	= 1 fluidounce (fl oz)
1 fluidounce	= 480 minims (m)
16 fluidounces	= 1 pint (pt, O)
2 pints (32 fluidounces)	= 1 quart (qt)
4 quarts (8 pints)	= 1 gallon (gal, C)

Measure of Weight

20 grains (gr)	= 1 scruple
3 scruples (60 grains)	= 1 dram
8 dram (480 grains)	= 1 ounce
12 ounces (5760 grains)	= 1 pound

Conversion Equivalents

1 g	= 15.432 gr
1 Kg	= 2.2 Avoirdupois lb
1 gr	= 0.0648 g or 64.8 or 65 mg
1 oz	= 31.1 g
1 oz (Avoir)	= 28.35 g, 437.5 gr
1 lb (Apoth)	= 373.2 g
1 lb (Avoir)	= 453.6 or 454 g, 16 oz
1 minim	= 0.06 ml
1 ml	= 16.23 minims
1 fl dr	= 3.69
1 fl oz	= 29.57 ml
1 pt	= 473 ml
1 gal (U.S.)	= 3785 ml
1 inch	= 2.54 cm
1 meter	= 39.37 inches

Fahrenheit to Centigrade	$-5(°F - 32)/9 = °C$ or $[(°F + 40) \times 5/a] - 40 = °C$
Centigrade to Fahrenheit	$-(°C \times 9)/5 + 32 = °F$ or $[(°C + 40) \times 9/5] - 40 = °F$
Centigrade to Kelvin	$-°C + 273 = °K$

ANATOMICAL
ILLUSTRATIONS

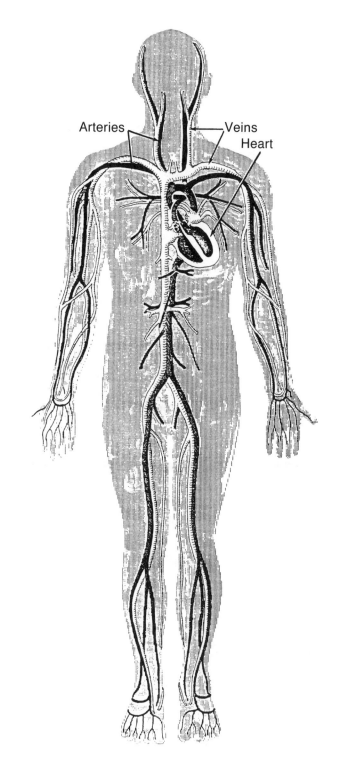

Arteries

Veins

Heart

CIRCULATORY SYSTEM

315

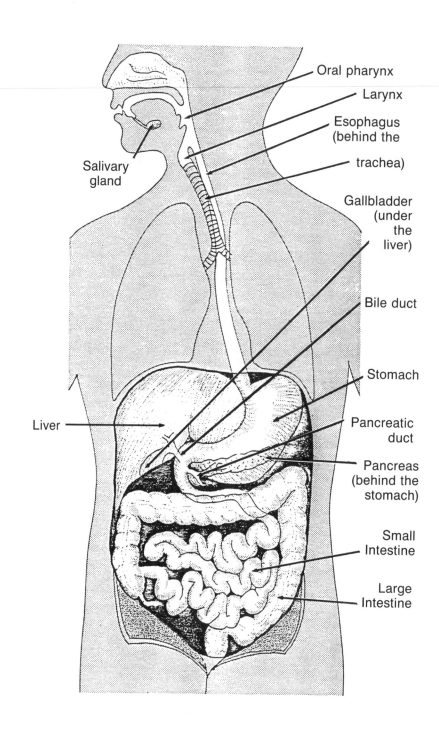

DIGESTIVE SYSTEM

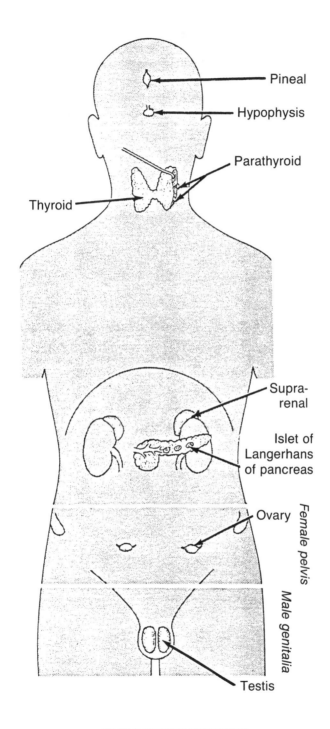

Pineal

Hypophysis

Parathyroid

Thyroid

Supra-renal

Islet of Langerhans of pancreas

Ovary

Female pelvis

Male genitalia

Testis

ENDOCRINE SYSTEM

317

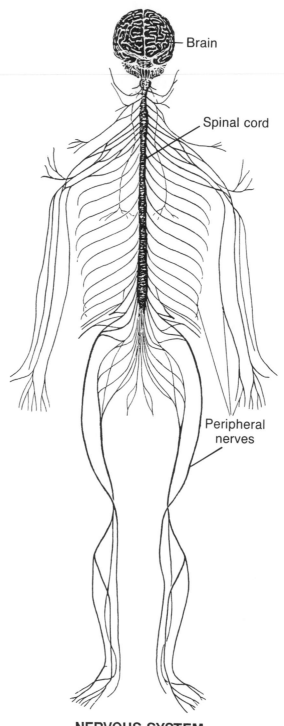

Brain

Spinal cord

Peripheral
nerves

NERVOUS SYSTEM

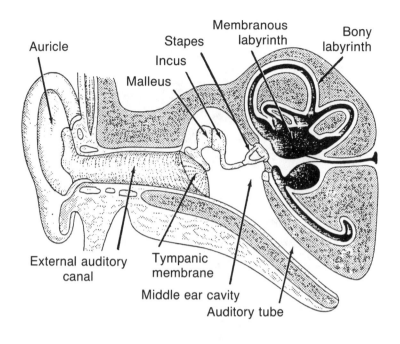

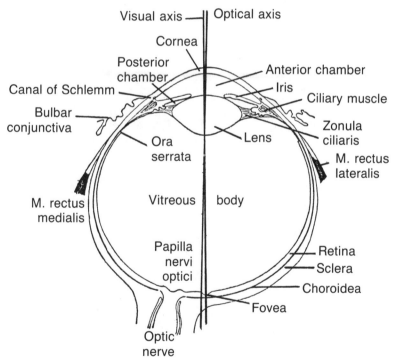

ORGANS OF SPECIAL SENSE

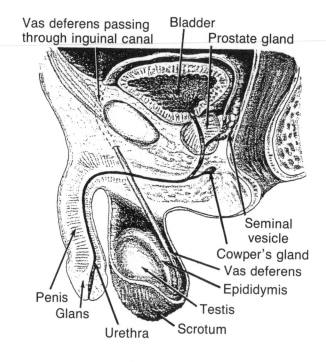

Vas deferens passing through inguinal canal

Bladder

Prostate gland

Seminal vesicle

Cowper's gland

Vas deferens

Epididymis

Penis

Glans

Testis

Urethra

Scrotum

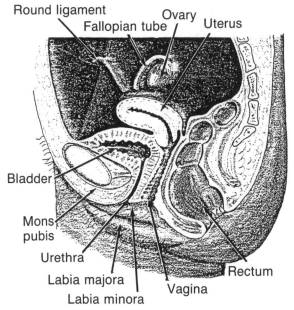

Round ligament

Fallopian tube

Ovary

Uterus

Bladder

Mons pubis

Urethra

Labia majora

Labia minora

Vagina

Rectum

REPRODUCTIVE SYSTEM

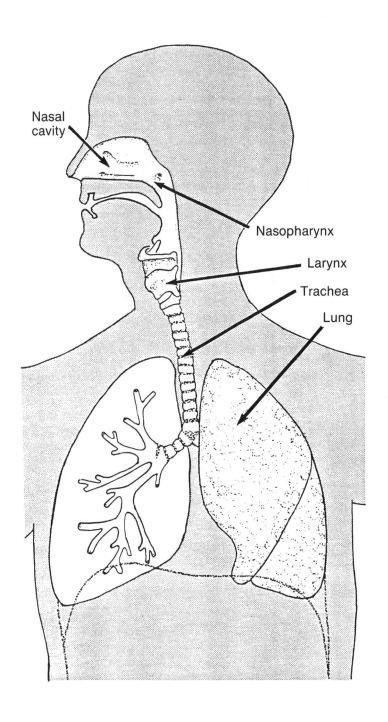

Nasal
cavity

Nasopharynx

Larynx

Trachea

Lung

RESPIRATORY SYSTEM

321

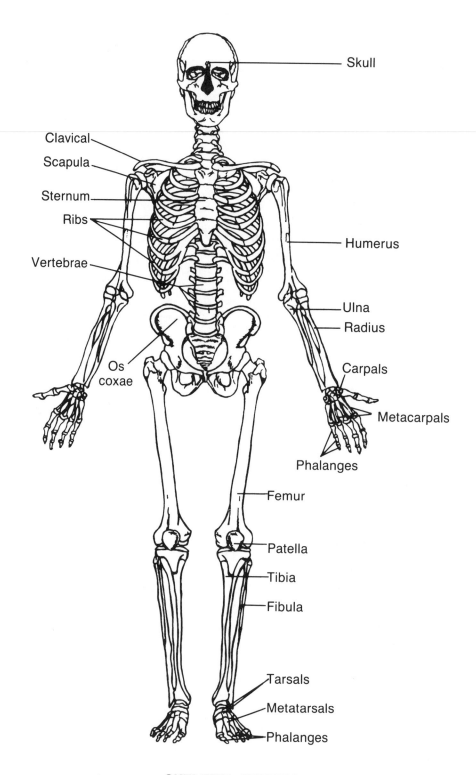

Skull

Clavical

Scapula

Sternum

Ribs

Vertebrae

Os coxae

Humerus

Ulna

Radius

Carpals

Metacarpals

Phalanges

Femur

Patella

Tibia

Fibula

Tarsals

Metatarsals

Phalanges

SKELETAL SYSTEM